The Nurse's Handbook of Spiritual Care

T0312705

The Nurse's Handbook of Spiritual Care

Pamela Cone

Azusa Pacific University, California, US

Tove Giske

VID Specialized University, Norway

WILEY Blackwell

Registered Offices
John Wiley & Sons, Inc., 111 River Street, Hoboken, NJ 07030, USA
John Wiley & Sons Ltd, The Atrium, Southern Gate, Chichester, West Sussex, PO19 8SQ, UK

Editorial Office
9600 Garsington Road, Oxford, OX4 2DQ, UK

For details of our global editorial offices, customer services, and more information about Wiley products visit us at www.wiley.com.

Wiley also publishes its books in a variety of electronic formats and by print-on-demand. Some content that appears in standard print versions of this book may not be available in other formats.

Library of Congress Cataloging-in-Publication Data applied for
[PB ISBN: 9781119890775]

Cover Design: Wiley
Cover Image: © Sandipkumar Patel/Getty Images

Set in 10.5/13pt STIXTwoText by Straive, Pondicherry, India

SKY10035598_080422

The authors dedicate this handbook on spiritual care to our parents, who taught us the way of living for Christ, and to our husbands, Dave and Jarl, who provided unwavering support to us for our research and writing. This book would not have been possible without you and your encouragement and that of our families. We thank God for you all!

Contents

Acknowledgements

The authors appreciate the support given by our home universities, Azusa Pacific University in California and VID Specialized University in Norway. Thank you for the encouragement from our leaders for our research and writing on spiritual care in nursing.

Preface

The Nurse's Handbook of Spiritual Care was developed for nursing students and nurses in all aspects of healthcare. The authors, an American nurse and a Norwegian nurse with 15 years of collaborative research, wrote a parallel book in Norwegian published in 2019 (*Å ta vare på heile mennesket: Handbok i åndeleg omsorg*) for the Scandinavian nursing audience. We hope this version, which presents a variety of European and American perspectives, will reach English-speaking nurses around the world. With this handbook, we want to help nurses develop competence as part of patient-centered, whole person care, and we want to show that spiritual care is a self-evident part of all nursing care. We would like to equip the reader with a professional perspective on this aspect of nursing care.

The authors build on extensive research in spiritual care by us as well as other nurse scholars interested in spirituality, and we present a learning spiral for improving knowledge and skills, which can lead to increased facility with spiritual care. By following the steps described, you can learn to "tune in" to patients and recognize and follow up on spiritual suffering and existential pain. You can also learn to use the inner resources that patients have for healing, and to reflect on/over the experience of what you have done to facilitate patient health and well-being. The purpose of this handbook is to motivate students and nurses and to improve their practice of spiritual and existential care as part of whole person healthcare.

All nursing education should teach spiritual care and ensure that students have fundamental knowledge, skills, and clinical practice within the spiritual domain so that they see this as an integral part of whole person or holistic nursing care. At the same time, supervisors in healthcare settings should ensure that the working environment is a welcoming one so that students and nurses can feel free to further develop their competence in this domain. Developing competencies for nurses can enable them to include data collection, situational assessment, follow-up, and reporting of patients' spiritual and/or existential needs and resources in their routine patient care.

Many colleagues have contributed to this project with ideas, tools, and stories. All of the examples used in this handbook are based on real events in the USA, Norway, and globally as reported by spiritual care researchers. Some come from our own practice and research, or they are stories from other scholarly research retold fully or in part, and edited to ensure the anonymity of patients, nurses, and students. Where we have used published narratives, we provide references. Together, these present a variety of resources that the readers can use to be inspired and challenged, and for reflection and learning. We use "patient" in this handbook knowing that some of the readers are nurses who utilize "clients" or "users."

The handbook covers the fundamentals of spiritual care so that reader awareness can be raised and nurses can be equipped and encouraged to open up and learn what the patients want to share with them. It is also important to emphasize that this is a field where no one is ever fully trained; there is always more to learn. All patients and situations you encounter are unique, and spiritual relationships can be expressed and met in a variety of ways. We will emphasize from the beginning the importance of life-long learning in this field. The handbook includes an introduction to the spiritual domain, followed by three chapters on the steps of preparing, connecting, and reflecting on the spiritual. Finally, we conclude with a chapter on self-care nursing with strategies to empower yourself and others in healthy ways. It also provides further discussions and resources to increase life-long learning of spiritual care.

The learning spiral, a teaching-learning theory developed by the authors in our early spiritual care research in Norway, is what guides the three chapters that follow. These chapters each deal with one of the three phases of the learning spiral. Chapters 2 through 4 are structured in the same way with an introduction to topics illustrated by stories that are followed by questions for reflection and suggestions for competencies that nurses can use.

Chapter 1 – *Basics of Spirituality and Spiritual Care* is a discussion of how spirituality and spiritual care are understood by the nursing profession globally. We begin with the premise that whole person care includes the physical, psychosocial, and spiritual. Spirituality is about existential questions; it is about meaning and purpose and hope as well as connectedness to self, others, and the transcendent. It addresses what a view of life is from different perspectives. It also includes religion and faith traditions with a variety of rituals and practices. We know that quality care is an important part of person-centered, whole person nursing care, and the ethical standards that guide the curriculum for nursing education, theory, practice, and research as well as the reporting and documentation of care represent a view of nursing care that includes spiritual care as an integral part of the nurse's area of responsibility.

Chapter 2 – *Preparing for Spiritual Care* is the first phase of the process. Initially, we go into different aspects of knowing yourself on a deeper level. We encourage the reader to consider why this is important in the exercise of spiritual care, and we invite the reader into various activities that can help in the process of becoming better acquainted with your own views, prejudices, attitudes, and stereotypes, particularly related to the spiritual domain. We also go through some assessment guides that can help nurses identify what patients need that is of a spiritual nature. Preparation is done through reading, reflecting, journaling, and dialoguing on the topic. At the end of the chapter, we look more closely at general and special competencies for spiritual care.

Chapter 3 – *Connecting: Recognizing and Following up on the Spiritual* discusses how we can identify, assess, and follow up on spiritual/existential and life-related situations and conditions with patients. We also address how to identify and use the patient's resources in the same way that we consider and follow up the physiological and psychosocial needs of patients for whom we are responsible. When there is something of a spiritual nature that is at stake in the patient's life, we illustrate the iterative process until he or she gets help. Scenarios and questions for reflection are integrated throughout the chapter. We discuss how to report spiritual needs and resources, and illustrate this with a story. The chapter concludes with a review of various factors that affect the spiritual care process.

Chapter 4 – *Reflecting on Experiences in Spiritual Care* is where we look more closely at how important reflection is for events and experiences to be transformed into growth and wisdom. We also look at how we can work with reflection both individually and in groups to deepen our understanding of what is spiritual in nature, what is considered as best practice in various situations, and how we can improve our patient-centered, whole person care. We go into what competencies students will develop during their course of study and how nurses can further develop competence in spiritual care as they encounter the deep inner spirit needs of patients.

Chapter 5 –*Life-long Learning and More* is where we discuss how nurses can grow and mature into healthy and robust professionals who thrive in any healthcare setting. We promote self-care of the nurse by focusing on how nurses can pay attention to our own needs and care for ourselves, thus avoiding burnout. Assertiveness training and development of a variety of coping strategies is discussed. We face head-on the challenge of bullying in the workplace and how caring for the spirit can counteract such negative practices among nurses. In this way, we will avoid the promotion of a hostile environment, and instead provide a warm and welcoming environment for patients and their families as well as for our fellow healthcare professionals. We conclude with more resources to promote increased capacity in and facilitation of spiritual care so that nurses can thrive in our challenging healthcare environment.

About the Authors

PAMELA CONE, PhD, RN, APRN-CNS, PHN
Professor, Masters & Doctoral Nursing Programs, School of Nursing, Azusa Pacific University, Azusa, CA USA

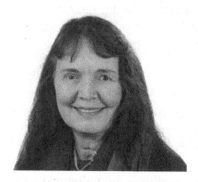

Dr. Pamela Cone was born and raised in Haiti by missionary parents and has been a nurse since 1974 and a nurse educator for 31 years. She has taught courses in theory, research, international health, and writing with bachelor, masters, and doctoral students at Azusa Pacific University and has served as an expert in Grounded Theory research for doctoral students since 2006. Her 2006 PhD dissertation was *Reconnecting: A Grounded Theory Study among Formerly Homeless Mothers*. A Fulbright Scholar in Norway in 2008-2009, Cone worked collaboratively with Norwegian Nurse Researcher, Dr. Tove Giske, to develop several grounded theories from their spirituality research. She was awarded the Beverly Hardcastle Stanford research grant from APU in 2014 for a semester of research in Norway. In collaboration with the EPICC scholars, their Spiritual Care Education and Practice (SEP) research team received a four-year Excellence in Research award from VID in Norway for research in spiritual care education and practice for

2020 through 2023, which is their current work. Together, Drs. Cone and Giske have edited two books as well as authoring two, published over a dozen articles in spirituality and spiritual care, and have presented their work in spiritual care education and practice at professional conferences and workshops in 25 countries to date around the world.

https://www.apu.edu/
https://discover.apu.edu/?s=School+of+Nursing+Faculty

TOVE GISKE, PhD, MPhil, RN
Professor, VID Specialized University Faculty of Health Studies Bergen, Norway

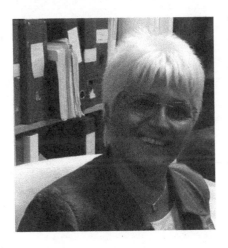

Tove Giske is a Professor in Nursing and works as a professor and researcher at VID Specialized University, Faculty of Health Studies, Bergen, where she also serves as the Director of Research and Development. She has researched and published widely internationally about spiritual care. She has collaborated with Professor Pamela Cone for over 20 years, and they have published a Handbook about Spiritual Care together in Norwegian (2019), and a similar English book in 2022. Tove has been a part of a European spiritual care network, which now has developed into the EPICC network, including the Spiritual care Education and Practice (SEP) Team that wrote the 4-year grant to develop materials in spiritual care for nurses and students globally. She developed an interest in how to serve nurses internationally and has been doing so since 1984. The last 4 years she has been the President of Nurses Christian Fellowship International and she seeks ways to teach and serve nurses around the world.

https://www.vid.no/en/employees/tove-giske/
https://app.cristin.no/persons/show.jsf?id=46926
https://www.researchgate.net/profile/Tove_Giske2

CHAPTER 1

Basics of Spirituality and Spiritual Care

WHAT IS SPIRITUAL CARE?

The authors asked that question during our 2008 study in Norway of how teachers understand and teach about care that is spiritual in nature. One teacher said this:

> I was working with students in the clinical setting at a nursing home where many patients had dementia. During our pre-conference time a student asked how the nurses could give spiritual care when the patients could not answer questions or talk about their beliefs and values. The nurse thought a moment and said, "I make waffles." The students looked at each other in puzzlement. "Waffles?" one said. "Yes, I make waffles, and you know, the patients are so happy to smell them and eat them, and they just love it! I don't know what they are thinking, but they are happy for a long time afterwards. So, yes, I make waffles."

The Nurse's Handbook of Spiritual Care, First Edition. Pamela Cone and Tove Giske.
© 2022 John Wiley & Sons Ltd. Published 2022 by John Wiley & Sons Ltd.

To contextualize this story, many Norwegians have a long tradition of having family time on Saturdays, with families gathering in the kitchen and making waffles with lots of delicious toppings. These are precious times for the family (families have various ways of preparing waffles that are passed down from mother to daughter), and this cultural practice is something that every Norwegian understands is important to the family. So, what made this waffle-making activity spiritual in nature? It certainly is not related to religion or faith, but rather, it is about something that touches what is deeply important to someone, what gives a person a sense of love and belonging, regardless of any ability to think or actually remember events.

In this chapter, we first present how spirituality and spiritual care are understood by the nursing profession and in relation to health globally. We discuss existential questions that often arise in situations of uncertainty or serious illness before we raise the issue of religion or faith tradition and what a view of life or life-view is. That spiritual care is part of the nurse's area of responsibility is evident in the ethical guidelines for nurses (ANA 2015; ICN, 2021) and in nursing theories like the Artinian Intersystem Model (Artinian et al. 2011; McEwen and Wills 2017) and Neuman's Systems Model (Alligood 2018; Petiprin 2016) that emphasize the central role of spirituality in every person.

The Artinian Intersystems Model (*AIM*) has a view of person that is threefold (biological, psychosocial, and spiritual) with spirituality at the core of the person (Artinian 1991). Nursing students at Azusa Pacific University (*APU*), where Artinian taught while developing her model, use this focus of person in their nursing care plans, requiring the nurse to complete assessments of all three aspects of the person. The focus of the AIM, with its traffic light framework for identifying knowledge (comprehensibility), values/beliefs/attitudes (meaningfulness), and behaviors/actions (manageability), is to assess the patient and the nurse in these areas and to develop a mutually negotiated plan of care (Artinian et al. 2011; McEwen and Wills 2017). By requiring regular spiritual assessment alongside the other domains, the nursing program heightens student awareness and understanding of the spiritual area. Spirituality is a thread that runs through the APU nursing curriculum from bachelors through doctoral studies.

The systems focus of Betty Neuman's model emphasizes the "wholistic" approach to nursing (Neuman 1996) and the openness required to appropriately gather information. The Neuman Systems Model (*NSM*) also identifies the spiritual as an integral part of the whole person (physiological, psychological, sociocultural, developmental, and spiritual), with all aspects of the core structure focused on basic survival factors that allow the human system to function (McEwen and Wills 2017). For Neuman, the spiritual variable includes beliefs and influences that provide lines of defense around the core of the person to help their spirit survive and thrive. The interrelationship between the five aspects of the person is crucial to appropriate functioning of the whole person. Neuman is also known for promoting three aspects of prevention (primary, secondary, and tertiary) that help the system work at peak efficiency (Alligood 2018). The NSM supports the importance of gathering information on spiritual resources of patients as well as identifying the needs, both met and unmet, in the spiritual realm that can help guide spiritual care.

The North American Nursing Diagnosis Association (NANDA 2016) addresses four elements of care that are spiritual in nature:

1. meaning and purpose, especially in light of health challenges
2. love and belonging (or connectedness and relationships to self, others, and the environment)
3. hope versus hopelessness or despair and
4. religious beliefs, values, and practices and/or faith traditions and a sense of the transcendent (Herdman and Kamitsuru 2017).

A person experiences spiritual well-being when those needs are met; but if any of those needs are not met, there can be spiritual distress (Herdman and Kamitsuru 2017; Taylor et al. 2019b). This is similar to the European understanding of nursing care that includes three elements of spirituality: meaning, connections, and transcendence (Kristofferson et al. 2016). Other theorists organize these components in different ways (McSherry and Ross 2010). Regardless of the definition of spirituality, spiritual care is an integral part of nursing care and an area of ethical responsibility of the nurse (ANA 2010).

Spirit – Breath of Life

In nursing literature, "the spirit" is understood in a broad sense as being the element that holds the person together, and though we have no common global definition of what it is all about, there is a general understanding that it is central to the person (Artinian et al. 2011; Stoll 1979; Taylor et al. 2019b). The spirit encompasses the entire human being and is not material or tangible. It is the intangible "breath of life" of every being. The spirit of a person touches on the inner being and may be expressed alone or when interacting with others. Spirituality includes the big questions in life, as well as peace of mind or inner peace, and is what provides the life spark of a human being. It is important for health and for the experience of wholeness in which body, soul, and spirit form the entire being (Rykkje 2016; Stoll 1979).

The authors of this handbook exemplify cultural diversity to some extent since we are from very different backgrounds. The first author is American (though born of missionary parents and raised in Haiti), living in the Los Angeles, California area where many cultures and people groups intersect, so a variety of views on the spiritual are regularly encountered by nurses. In contrast, the word for "spiritual" in the Norwegian context, where our second author lives, has a religious overtone that causes people to think immediately of faith, religion, and Christianity, which she sees as too narrow for a multicultural global society. In areas where spirituality is entwined with religious or faith-based meanings, some nurses would rather use the word "existential," which has a broad non-religious meaning. Because the nature of spirituality is interpreted differently across countries and cultures around the world, it can be difficult to grasp and hard to explain.

In light of this lack of consensus, we present various views, descriptions, and definitions of the spiritual as understood by nurses in a variety of settings. At times, we use the concepts spiritual and existential together (spiritual/existential) to encourage a broad understanding of spirituality.

The English nursing association, the Royal College of Nursing (*RCN*), defines spirituality as being about hope and strength, trust, goals and thinking, empathy, beliefs and values, love and relationships, morality, creativity, and being able to express yourself and communicate with others (RCN 2011). These are many keywords that go back to what the spiritual is across nursing literature. The RNC created a nurse pocket guide as a free download to help address spiritual issues as part of nursing care (www.rcn.org.uk).

Another way of discussing spirituality is in the European Association of Palliative Care (*EAPC*) literature, where scholars provide a consensus definition for this concept. "Spirituality is the dynamic dimension of human life that relates to the way people (individual and community) experience, express and/or seek meaning, purpose and transcendence, and the way they connect to the moment, to self, to others, to nature, to the significant and/ or to the sacred" (Nolan et al. 2011, p. 88). Within their definition, spirituality encompasses three primary dimensions:

1. existential questions (concerning, for example, identity, meaning, suffering and death, guilt and shame, reconciliation and forgiveness, freedom and responsibility, hope and despair, and love and joy)
2. value-based considerations and attitudes (that is, the things most important to each person, such as relations to oneself, family, friends, work, things, nature, art and culture, ethics and morals, and life itself)
3. religious considerations and foundations (faith, beliefs and practices, rituals, one's relationship with God or the ultimate) (Nolan et al. 2011, p. 88).

Additionally, an Irish research team analyzed 47 theoretical and empirical articles from various areas to clarify the content of the concept of spirituality (Weathers et al. 2016). The analysis shows that the spirit has many dimensions, the individual person has a unique history, and the spirit is expressed in different ways among different people. The relationship aspect encompasses the self and attachment to others, the environment and/or nature, and/or a higher power or something that is beyond self, together with a sense of meaning in life. Another aspect of the spirit is the experience of transcendence beyond yourself, everyday life, and the world in which you live. Transcendence is the ability to transform or change perspective on a given situation or life in general so that the experience of the situation changes and moves beyond self. Weathers et al. (2016) found three defining attributes of spirituality: acknowledgement of a higher power or someone/something beyond self; connections or attachment/relationship to self, others, and nature; and the need to find meaning and purpose in life. Transcendence, relationship, and meaning are thus found across nursing literature, and the importance of caring for patients spiritually as part of whole person, patient-centered care is in most foundational nursing textbooks (Kristofferson et al. 2016; Taylor et al. 2019b).

We summarize the spiritual domain with a paraphrased narrative from psychiatrist Victor Frankl, a holocaust survivor who wrote *Man's Search for Meaning* (Frankl 1946/1959).

> *A widower came to Frankl for treatment. After his wife's death, the man felt that life was no longer worth living. Over time, this man and the psychiatrist talked about many different things, and during one conversation, Frankl asked him, "What would it be like if you were the one who died and your wife the one who lived as a widow?" "Oh," said the man, "that would not be good! If it were one of us who had to die first, it was good that I'm the one who lived, because I am better able to live alone than she would be."*

This extract from Frankl's conversations with the widower highlights the importance of having meaning in relationships and finding what is meaningful for each of us. The man had felt that his life no longer had meaning since he was alone. The question about what it would have been like if he had been the one who died, and thus, avoiding a life with such great sadness, made him suddenly look at his situation with new awareness. Thus the whole experience of the situation changed (transcendence), and he had a new sense of purpose for his grief (meaning), namely, that he had saved his wife from the experience of being widowed and living alone.

Reflection 1.1

- After reading the different ways of describing "the spirit," what do you think about "the spirit" in your own life?
- How would you define or describe the spiritual domain?
- What element of the spiritual do you see most often when caring for others?
- Do you recognize spiritual expressions, cues, or themes when working with patients?

SPIRITUAL CARE

What then is spiritual care? Spiritual care can be summed up as caring for the whole person through patient-centered care and being completely present for the other, by listening for what is important in the patient's life, and often by facilitating practical matters that are deeply important to the person (Carson 2011; Kuven and Bjørvatn 2015; Rykkje 2016; Taylor et al. 2019b). American nurse philosopher and theorist Jean Watson (1997) has presented many spiritual aspects of care in her *10 Caritas Factors* (Watson 1999; Wei and Watson 2011) that are foundational to caring practice in nursing.

1) humanistic and altruistic values; 2) faith/hope; 3) sensitivity to self/others; 4) developing helping, trusting, caring relationships; 5) accepting/expressing positive/negative feelings/emotions; 6) creative/individualized/problem-solving; 7) transpersonal teaching/learning; 8) supportive, protective, or corrective mental/physical/societal/spiritual environment; 9) human needs helping; and 10) phenomenological existential, or spiritual forces

(Alligood 2018, pp. 95–96).

Of these factors, more than half explicitly address the spiritual (1–5, 8, and 10), while others (6, 7, and 9) have a more implicit connection to the inner person/spirit. These remind us that compassionate care comes from the inner spirit of the nurse.

Danish nurse researcher Vibecke Østergaard Steenfeldt puts it this way: "Spiritual care is to have the courage to go with the patient into the space of the suffering and be there with the patient" (Steenfeldt et al. 2018, p. 34). The purpose of spiritual care it is "to help the patient with life development" (p. 30). Spiritual care alleviates patient suffering and increases a sense of well-being and of feeling supported (Best et al. 2015). When life is difficult, the spiritual can be an important resource, which can help the patient achieve a sense of inner peace and strength (Giske and Cone 2015; Rykkje 2016; Taylor et al. 2019b; Weathers et al. 2016). Spiritual health promotion is part of whole person nursing care and includes relieving or alleviating pain and/or suffering, or simply treating the patient with dignity and respect. Jessie, a patient who was very anxious to go home the day after having a stroke, haltingly told the nurse this story:

I had a stroke on my right side, and the night nurse put the call button on that side even though my hand is weak. During the night, I had to use the toilet, but I couldn't press the button. I tried calling out, but nobody came. I tried to hold my urine, but finally, I could not, so I wet the bed. I felt so humiliated! I lay there for a long time in a wet bed until morning when that nurse came to check on things near the end of her shift. She said to me "You all right, honey? Oh, you peed in the bed! Oh dear, I guess we'll have to put a diaper on you!" I said "Sorry!" but she did not answer. She came back with another nurse and proceeded to change the bed, just rolling me from side to side and talking over my head to the other nurse, and then putting a big diaper on me and settling me down again with the call light still by my weak right hand! She never called me by name, just "honey" and she never found out that I can hold my urine just fine as long as I get a bedpan when I need it!

The day shift nurse, who had listened patiently while Jessie struggled to communicate, apologized for the way her inner sense of dignity was destroyed and her spirit was hurt by the night nurses' attitudes and actions. The nurse removed the diaper and made Jessie comfortable again, and then placed the call light beside her strong left hand.

Reflection 1.2

- What was spiritual about this nurse-patient encounter?
- What would have changed this encounter into a positive, uplifting experience?
- How did the day nurse provide spiritual care?
- Can you think of a time when practical care had/has a spiritual dimension to it?

The RCN in the UK also made a list of what kind of care is *not* spiritual. According to these guidelines, spiritual care is not simply about religious beliefs and practices; such needs can be referred to the appropriate spiritual leader. Nor is it right for students or nurses to force their personal values on a captive audience, threaten others with their own beliefs, or exploit situations to persuade patients to change their beliefs to match those of the nurse, all of which are completely unethical (Fowler 2020). Spiritual care is not just a responsibility for specialists or especially interested nurses, and it is not simply the responsibility of the hospital chaplain/priest or other religious leaders (ANA 2010; RCN 2011).

Spiritual care is about being interested in and paying attention to the patient's deep inner concerns and/or existential questions (Cone 2020). By encouraging the patient to express himself or herself and listening in an open and non-judgmental way to the patient sharing his/her own beliefs and traditions, the nurse is providing supportive spiritual care. Moreover, spiritual care is about how one carries out practical and concrete nursing care, that is a combination of what we do (the science of nursing) and the way we do it (the art of nursing), both of which are very important (Cone 2020; Taylor et al. 2019a). Spiritual competencies include knowledge, skills, and attitudes as we provide care (Van Leeuwen and Cusveller 2004). It can be about how we wash and feed a patient, change dressings on wounds, or change the diaper on a patient who is incontinent. The way these things are performed can alleviate suffering, build good relationships, and strengthen hope in a patient, or it can increase suffering and lessen hope and life courage, which is the courage to be (Clark 2013).

With patients and their families in clinical practice, we seek to understand the patient's situation in a whole person way rather than dividing things up to consider physical, mental, emotional, social, and spiritual elements separately; all of these are interwoven in a human being's life (McSherry and Ross 2010). During the learning process, it may still be necessary to clarify that spiritual care has its own characteristics that you can consciously look for, read about, discuss within the nursing profession, and report on or document. However, as you grow in your understanding, whole person care will begin to weave these elements all back together (Cone 2020). In the work to develop quality of life goals for spirituality, religiousness, and personal beliefs, the World Health Organization conducted a large, 18-country international study in 2002 and developed eight characteristics that distinguish spiritual care from psychosocial care (WHO-QOL SRPB Group 2006). They found that quality of life that measures spirituality, religion, and personal faith is about:

1. what relationship one has to a spiritual being or power and how it helps one through difficult times and stress

2. the meaning of life, which is related to the experience of meaning, if one feels that one has a goal or purpose in life, and whether one feels that one has a reason to live

3. to what extent one experiences awe in relation to nature, music, art, or beauty and whether one experiences being grateful

4. wholeness and integration, which is about the experience of the relationship between mind, body, and soul and consistency between thoughts and feelings

5. spiritual strength, which relates to the extent to which the inner spirit helps one to bear it when life is difficult as well as helping one to be happy in life

6. inner peace/calm/harmony, which is about to what degree one has inner peace and feels an inner harmony with oneself

7. hope and optimism, seeking hope or being hopeful and optimistic in life and

8. to what extent faith contributes to well-being, strength, and joy in life (WHO-QOL SRPB Group 2006).

Spiritual care is not just about addressing spiritual needs; it also includes helping the patient access spiritual resources that bring joy and strength, thus helping them not only to survive but also to thrive (Cone 2020). The National Health Service (*NHS*) Education in Scotland, which has worked extensively with what kind of care is spiritual in nature and what space it should have in healthcare, describes spiritual care as care that:

> . . .*recognizes and responds to the need of man's spirit. . . Spiritual care can include the need for self-worth, for expressing, for support, perhaps for ritual or prayer or sacrament, or just for a sensitive listener. Spiritual care begins with encouraging human contact in a compassionate relationship and moves in the direction needed.*
>
> (NHS 2009, p. 6)

The last part of the quote, *moves in the direction needed*, means that the patient is the one who decides what is important

(Giske and Cone 2015). It is not the nurse controlling the process; the nurse should follow the patient on the path they or their family need. We must be willing to go where the patient is and at the pace the patient sets (Giske and Cone 2015; Minton et al. 2018). *Journeying with* (Cone and Giske 2013b) can mean following along with or being a fellow human being together on a learning journey or on a mutual journey through crisis and suffering (Cone and Giske 2013a, 2013b; Edwards et al. 2016; Krauss et al. 2016).

Reflection 1.3

- After reading all this, what is your understanding of spiritual care?
- How are the spiritual and psychological similar when giving care?
- In what ways are the spiritual, psychological, and/or social different?
- What do you think is important about distinguishing between spiritual and psychosocial care?

THE SPIRITUAL AS PART OF WHOLE PERSON CARE

The spiritual is an integral part of whole person nursing care (Taylor et al. 2019a). Humanity is body, soul, and spirit at the same time, so while we meet as physical human beings with personalities, cultures, attitudes, and experiences, there is also a spiritual encounter. The Norwegian nursing education plan for mental health (Norwegian Ministry of Health and Care [NMHC] 2009) emphasizes that existential questions and spiritual expressions must be seen as an integral part of health services:

> *A person with mental problems must not only be seen as a patient, but as a whole person with body, soul and spirit.*

Necessary considerations must be taken of human spiritual and cultural needs, not just the biological and the social. Mental disorders affect basic existential issues and this must characterize the construction, practice and management of all health services.

(NMHC 2009, State Proposition 63, p. 6)

The spiritual is not always clear, since humans are integrated creatures who cannot be limited to a particular aspect or area; spirituality can only be understood together with everything else in a human being's life. One patient who was asked if he experienced spiritual care while he was hospitalized replied: "Yes, I did, but I do not believe that the one giving it was aware of it." This may also be true in the following story of another nurse-patient encounter.

A nursing student in clinical practice at a stroke unit worked with Anna, who had right-side paralysis in the right hand and foot as well as in the throat so she could not eat or drink and had lost the ability to talk. Anna was clear and oriented and could write left-handed on a tablet what she wanted or needed. It came out clearly, both in body language and in the words written on the tablet, that she was feeling down. Anna felt bothered because she needed a lot of help. The student, who cared for Anna together with many different nurses, saw that the nurses treated Anna with care and respect. This showed in the way they cared for, talked with, and worked with her on her treatments. One of the nurses said that it was important for Anna to have a good time and that she had chosen to work at a stroke unit because she liked this work. Both Anna and the student knew that these words went from heart to heart. That nurse gave Anna a hug and Anna cried – and she was allowed to cry. When the student reflected on what she had learned in this clinical placement, the student said: "Real care builds up human dignity!"

Reflection 1.4

- What do you think of the claim that a person is "spirit, and when you meet a fellow human being, there is a spiritual encounter"?
- What do you think about spiritual care in the story of Anna?
- Can you think of a time when you may have provided spiritual care without realizing it?

EXISTENTIAL QUESTIONS

In the literature on spiritual care, existential and religious needs and resources are usually addressed separately. Existential longing and existential questions are general, and we find them expressed in philosophy and in religions related to questions such as "What gives life meaning?", "Why am I suffering?", "What can I do with my guilt?", and "What happens after death?" In the face of illness, crisis, loss, and/or impending death, these questions surface more readily than when life goes on in a normal fashion.

When the existential quest and longing, or even pain, awakens within, it touches the innermost part of a person. What we have to help us is our philosophy of life, our successes in life, our own life story of good and bad experiences, as well as the people around us – family, friends, and professional helpers. Knowledge of mental and physical health, different forms of treatment, and social networking is not contrary to knowledge of existential longing, but it helps us to see the context and thus gives a complementary picture of the patient's situation. Existential wonder, questions, or pain is a general spiritual phenomenon that touches us all whether we are nurses or patients.

Reflection 1.5

- What gives you a sense of meaning in life? How do you create meaning in your life?

- What makes you feel a sense of security or of freedom?
- What do you do with the experience of emotional and/or existential doubt?
- What do you think will happen when you die? What is beyond this life?
- Have you encountered existential questions in others?
- If you have met this in others, what did you learn that you can take with you in life for your professional experience?

In one research interview, a nursing student we will call Marta reflected on how breaking both bones in her right forearm as a 12-year-old changed her future:

When I was 12 years old, my great passion was playing handball. I talked about playing on the national team; Norway had the world's best women's handball team! Then I was unlucky and broke both bones in my right forearm in a bad fall. Nurses and doctors at the hospital talked to my parents about the injury and treatment and explained that healing would come with time. The nurses were pleasant, but no one talked to me about the injury and the healing process. At night, I thought that I would never be able to play handball again and was very sad because I had to give up the big dream of my life. None of the nurses asked me why I was sad; they just feared that I was in pain and they thought I was a quiet and withdrawn child because I did not talk about my arm. I worked through this loss and grief all alone and cried my tears quietly in the pillow so no one could see it, and I never played handball again.

Several years later, when I thought about what I was going to be and how I should educate myself, I thought of the nurses I met as a 12-year-old in the hospital. Although they had not spoken to me, they had treated me with kindness and care, and I decided to become a nurse. During my early nursing education, I realized that with physiotherapy I could have trained my poor right arm to regain its full function and still become a professional handball player. Maybe I could have reached my dreams, if I had gotten better follow-up when I was a child! I wonder?

Reflection 1.6

- What existential themes do you recognize in Marta's story?
- How could the nurses have discovered what Marta was struggling with and sad about?
- What would you have done in this situation to help the child Marta?

RELIGION, RITUALS, AND FAITH PRACTICES

Religion comes from the Latin *religare*, which suggests to be bound to someone (Aadnanes 2012). To have a religious belief is to believe that there are other forms of existence or powers than what we can grasp with reason, see, or sense around us. Religions can be mainstream faith traditions or unique sets of beliefs held by people groups; they can also be defined in relation to categories of mythos, culture, and ethos (Aadnanes 2012; Bråten and Everington 2018). *Mythos* is the educational side of religion and communicates how one should understand God and humanity's place, tasks, and responsibilities in our existence. Culture relates to the social part of religious practice and can be understood through symbols and rituals when they bring together the divine and fellowship with others. *Ethos* is about values, moral norms, and practical ways of life that provide guidance for how to live (Aadnanes 2012).

Being religious is one way of being spiritual where the religion provides an interpretive framework in the face of big questions about life and death (Chan et al. 2006). American psychologist Kenneth Pargament raises another aspect of religion, namely the *sacred* (Pargament 2007). What is sacred to a person is not just about God. It is about every aspect of life that becomes extraordinary because of an affiliation with what is beyond self or represents transcendence for the person. It includes what is deeply personal and important to the patient that is sometimes hard to put into words. Understanding who/what is sacred to someone can help us to avoid violating patients; it can help us show respect even when we disagree.

Religions also have some type of organized structure in common. Because of a thousand-year history of Christianity in Norway (Catholic in the 1000s changing to Lutheran in the 1500s), there are values that have influenced societal views, and there is one large church organization along with many smaller religious groups. The Lutheran Church, which at one time was the State Church, makes up about 69% of the population, while other Christian groups together make up about 8% and other religions add up to about 5% of Norwegians, making 82% who have some type of religious beliefs, rituals, and/or practices (Statistics Norway 2019). Because many Norwegians were christened and confirmed or grew up in a church, people often know special music or hymns from a faith tradition when they, to a greater or lesser extent, interpret life in light of the doctrine of their childhood religion. They may actively participate in rituals and social activities and live in alignment with the values and norms of that religion, or they may simply have an underlying belief system with very limited actual practice of traditional rituals.

While there is no primary church in the United States, Christianity is also the largest religion in America, where 63% belong to some type of Christian church (both Catholic and Protestant Christian) organization, while 14% have some other faith or belief in God. This has declined about 8% in the last 7 years and varies about 10 percentage points among states, with Alabama being the most oriented to Christianity and Florida being the least, but overall, at least 77% of Americans have a religious belief of some kind (Pew Research Center [PRC] 2021). Percentages vary elsewhere in the world, but religion is a strong force globally. Because of this, nurses need to be able to determine if patients have a spiritual issue that has its roots in religion, and to either allow patients to express their concerns while simply listening attentively or to call in an appropriate spiritual leader to help them.

As nurses, we meet many patients who have a religious belief, and we have to defer our own beliefs while being open to supporting patients with different religious understandings from us. It is important to have good basic knowledge about different religions and health beliefs and about religious matters that are important in the face of illness and death (Fowler et al. 2011; Horsfjord 2017; Taylor 2012). We emphasize that what feels like a threat to an individual is not necessarily so when compared to our own views or to the mythos, culture, or ethos of a particular religion.

It is important that we, in addition to listening to what the patient says and identifying any existential issues that are emerging, also ask for the beliefs and values the patient holds. Without knowing how patients who have a religious belief seek to understand their life and can gain hope and strength through prayer, holy texts, fellowship, or other religious elements, it is difficult to facilitate and support the sacred in their care. The three following examples show how varying challenges that patients face can be woven into their life and can have decisive significance for nursing care. The first scenario is about a Muslim family.

This man, let's call him Hassan, had come from Afghanistan some years ago, and both he and his wife spoke Norwegian well and had many friends locally. This was a family with three young children when he got sick with cancer. Hassan was a devoutly practicing Muslim, and he and his wife often prayed for him to recover. He said that Allah's plan for life has no direct control over man, so the family tried to live day to day as best they could. Hassan went through a lot of treatment. He was optimistic with a cheerful and calm temperament and was sure he would get well.

But the cancer spread throughout Hassan's body and even metastasized to the brain, and the situation was difficult for everyone. His wife was tired, and Hassan was very scared and would have preferred to be home. Hassan was hospitalized and wished his wife would be there all the time to help with his care, something that was difficult with three young children at home. When the family couldn't be there, the nurses did their best to make sure Hassan got kind and humane care.

Many practicing Muslims were interacting more often when he was doing poorly and as death was approaching. Adherents visited and recited prayers and verses from the Quoran or Koran to him. Hassan also got a visit from an Imam, who prayed for him. Nurses placed the bed so that it stood in a way that made him face toward Mecca so he could pray whenever he wanted. Hassan had lots of visits, something that was important to him and his wife. Nurses did their best to facilitate important cultural values to Hassan and his family.

His wife was with Hassan when he was dying, and all the relatives they wanted were allowed to stay there in the room after his death. Hassan's wife took responsibility for the religious rituals that were important to them and gave comfort to the family, and the staff made sure that they were able to do all that they wanted to do.

Here we can recognize the three defining attributes of spirituality that were shown earlier: transcendence, relationships, and search for meaning (Weathers et al. 2016). We also see that facilitating rituals in relation to prayer was of great importance to this patient. For the wife and extended family and friends he would leave behind, ritual around the death was very important.

The second example illustrates that, even for patients who have dementia, beliefs can have great significance. In this story, the right to find peace in relation to what will happen to you after death is at stake. When the ability to put their thoughts and feelings into words is reduced, it adds an extra challenge for the nurse to interpret the patient's situation and find ways to help. One nurse shared the following experience with a Christian patient.

I had the evening shift in a nursing home and one of my patients was an elderly man we will call Ben who had dementia. I found Ben in a day care room, partly undressed and very agitated. Ben looked at me and asked, "Is there room for me?" Room for me, I thought, and there was something in the situation that made me wonder what was in this question. My thoughts went to Jesus' story in John's Gospel where He says to His disciples that they should not be afraid and that there are many rooms in His Father's house. Was this what Ben was wondering about more than what rooms he had here in the nursing home? "Is it heaven you are thinking of?" I asked to find out how I was going to move on in the conversation to help him. "YES!" Ben said, looking at me. "Do you know Jesus?" I asked. "YES!" he said again. I said, "The Bible says that all who receive Jesus have a place in heaven." Ben listened and became calm. "There is room for you," I confirmed. I followed Ben back to his room, and he found rest in bed.

The last example is a longer narrative of a foreign student who was studying nursing in a different country. He talked about meeting a patient in a nursing home who was seen by staff as very demanding. In addition, the student felt that it was difficult to relate to the patient's documented view of life since it was quite different from his own.

This elderly patient we will call Jacob had struggled with chronic pain and was bedridden. Jacob had poor vision and was very hard of hearing, something that made communication difficult. The staff had told me that Jacob was very Christian, often crying out loud to God when he was upset, angry, or in pain. They suggested I overlook this behavior because Jacob was deeply concerned with religious things. Jacob also had some routines that were very important to him, such as the Bible and hymn book should be in a special place on the nightstand. During the summer, I had enough experience with Jacob to share the staff's frustration

*with him, and it annoyed me that placing both the Bible
and the hymn book in exactly the right spot could take up to
20 minutes. And I was used to him calling for God, salva-
tion, Jesus, and Mary.*

*One day Jacob had been calling for a long time. I looked in
on him through the open door and didn't want to go inside.
All the others were busy, and Jacob was waving to me.
I reluctantly entered. I bent down to Jacob who nodded and
waved at the books on the nightstand. "No, please, no!"
A voice inside me said, "Not the books!" I pointed at the
black-bound Bible with gilded edges. Jacob shook his head.
I pointed at the dark brown book beside it. Jacob nodded
vigorously. He grabbed the book from me and tried to scroll
through it. I was a little surprised because I had expected a
long session to place the books in relation to the edge of the
bedside table. The brown book was old and well-used. What
I thought was a hymn book was full of biblical texts, one for
each day of the week. "So practical," I thought. I browsed
until Tuesday and read the text of the day.*

*Jacob grabbed my hand hard and nodded gratefully. He
did not protest when I put the book back on the bedside
table. He didn't see me going after it was closed. I went out,
almost a little disappointed that the whole thing was over so
fast. I looked around in the hallway. Was there anyone who
had seen or heard me? I looked at the clock; it had taken
just five minutes. And I had been both annoyed and a little
scared of the brown book. Small, precious words in an ordi-
nary evening. Special words that I had not planned for my
lips to shape or for my voice to say. It was just such a shame,
I thought, that Jacob could not read it for himself.*

*Several months later, I was on this same ward. I stopped in
the patient's doorway even though Jacob had not called.
Everyone knew he didn't have a long time left. I went in
and over to the bed. Jacob lay there quietly, and then he
reached out to grab my hand. His hands folded around*

mine, and he pleaded "please, please." I had heard in the report that Jacob had asked more of the staff to help him to let go. It was nagging at me. Was this what he asked me to do, did he plead for help to die? I understood, but I didn't want to think about what Jacob had, the pain that he had to endure.

Jacob pointed at the two books. He raised two folding hands. Then it hit me. Maybe he was asking for prayer! I browsed in the brown book I had read before, but found no prayers there. I was stressed and embarrassed by my own inability to help him. A dying patient is entitled to something more than this, I thought. Anything better than a foreign student! I thought of my godly childhood. I think pretty much Psalms and prayers in my own native language came to mind. The Lord's Prayer! The inspiration was like a light went off. I leaned over Jacob and shouted in his deaf ear: "Our Father who art in heaven, hallowed be Thy name. . ." His hair got into my nostrils. It was very unpleasant. I didn't feel anything about what I said. I screamed in discomfort at a god I do not know, but in a pattern the patient recognized. Then I realized Jacob was expressing his feelings. He lay there with pain, in darkness and isolation. I had cried out to God on his behalf.

"Amen." The word was spit out in a sigh of relief. Jacob released his grip on my arm and lay quietly. This time, I did not look around when I walked out of the room. I didn't care if anyone had heard. I had just called out a poor prayer, in a foreign language, for blind eyes and deaf ears. Afterwards, I wish Jacob could have told me why the prayer helped, though he had become calm. What is the secret of the sacred? Perhaps the answer is that no prayer is poor. There is no language that is foreign to God. And a prayer's effect is not dependent on whether it is believed by the nurse or heard by a deity; we just know it is said. For Jacob, shouting, and spitting God's name was a relief. As health *workers, we must learn to look beyond our own reactions to such expressions and work our way through our patients' different beliefs. Then we can actually help the patient express the need, regardless of how it feels to us.*

This example challenges us to think about how workplace cultures can evolve differently so that you might overlook or ignore patients' expressions of spiritual pain rather than addressing them. The story encourages us to reflect on whether exercising spiritual care saves time and/or if there are any times when not addressing patient spiritually can be acceptable. It also reminds us that there are spiritual resources a patient can use if we are willing to help the patient access them.

Reflection 1.7

- How can the nurse/student find out what the patient needs in these three situations?
- In what way is Jacob's situation different from the other scenarios?
- Think about what the nurse/student says in each scenario. How can what we learn from them have an influence on spiritual care that we facilitate?
- How would you meet these three patients?

Many of those who have a religious belief are not interested in being part of an organized faith community. They live out their faith in their own way. This form of private religion seems to be increasing in many areas. Often, people who are members of some major religion are not active participants and have little contact with church or temple outside of baptism, confirmation, marriage, and burial, and perhaps they go to church at Christmas, Easter, or some other religious holiday. Such a privatized faith often has little obvious acknowledgment and represents a voice that is almost silent in the public space. Personal belief is shaped by upbringing, background, and culture (Torskenæs et al. 2015). During crisis and illness, it may be important to understand this belief because it is what the patient uses to work through whatever is difficult in life. It is this, more than official doctrines of a particular religion, that is important for the nurse to understand.

In our spiritual care research, many patients we interview say something like, "I do not go to church and do not read in the Bible [or other sacred texts]." However, the family may have had some faith tradition in their childhood that has influenced them in some way. Others follow specific rituals related to their religion, such as prayer and dietary restrictions, but do not actually attend the church or temple, while still others gain spiritual strength from nature or a vague sense of the transcendent. Depending on what kind of beliefs people have, many turn to God with prayers when they face challenging life situations even if they never think about God in everyday life (Giske 2010). Rykkje et al. (2013) found in their study of the elderly that when death approaches, many people experience an increased need for religious support, and that childhood beliefs drilled into them throughout their early years once again became important to them. Nonjudgmentally helping patients to express their deeply held beliefs can be very healing.

Reflection 1.8

- Do you belong to any organized faith community?
- If so, to what extent do you share mythos, culture, and ethos that this community stands for?
- To what extent do you fit under the term "private beliefs"?
- What life experiences and understandings in relation to truth or faith are important to you?
- What can your experience mean for your understanding of and care for patients?

LIFE-VIEW

So, is spiritual care the same as religious care? What about those who are not religious? The Norwegian concept of life-view can help us with this concern. A view of life is a more or less coherent and theoretically understood reason for the terms, tasks, goals, and meaning of life human beings identify and use to function in society (Great Norwegian Lexicon 2017). One's outlook can be either religious or non-religious or even both. Not everyone is religious, but everyone has a view of life. This life-view is the sum of thoughts and beliefs we use to encounter and work with the big questions in life.

A life-view gives us perspective and frames how we understand the world in which we live. Through rituals and ceremonies, we come to understand the existence of life; moreover, the clearest situation to gauge the reality of one's view/perception of life is when life itself is at stake and/or when death is approaching. The way in which the dying person and the family move toward death, what happens to the dead after he or she is dead, and how to carry out a burial and follow the person's wishes, express what we believe is true about the life and the world we see and the one we do not see.

The life-view can be understood on two levels. The first level is about doctrines from a philosophy of life, similar to what we call mythos in religion. The second relates to how the individual experiences and integrates his or her view of life and interprets others' lives. In the same way as with religions, a life-view is on the personal plane where the work of finding context, understanding, and reaching acceptance happens. This work can take time and proceed at a slow pace for both patients and nurses, but having a reflected life-view is important because it can be useful and healing. For a nurse, it is very helpful to have a conscious relationship with his or her own view of life. A nurse who knows and is confident in what she or he believes can more easily collaborate with others and distinguish between personal values and points of view and what the patient's or family's life-view is; therefore, self-awareness is crucial for the nurse.

Having a reflected life-view does not necessarily mean having answers to all the patients' questions, but being confident in personal beliefs and aware of doubts can be helpful and allow us to be open hearted and open minded about differences. It enables us to treat our patients and their families with respect and dignity and to acknowledge that we do not have all the answers but that we are fully present with the patient. Also, being familiar with the typical questions a patient facing various crises might struggle with allows the nurse to be open and respectful of the patient's journey through suffering (Leenderts 2014).

Reflection 1.9

- Can you put your view of life into words?
- What is a person's responsibility and task in life?
- How do you understand life, suffering, and death?
- What do you think is the value of having a reflective life-view?

WHY SPIRITUAL CARE IS IMPORTANT IN NURSING CARE

To answer this question about the importance of spiritual care in nursing, we are assisted by the German psychiatrist and philosopher Karl Jaspers (1883–1969), who wrote that humans are always in situations (Gatta 2015). Each situation unfolds in a specific place, at a given time, and with one or more people involved. Situations can be influenced and changed by many things (Gatta 2015; Wikström 2001). We can decide if we want to go out with friends one evening or stay home, whether we want to do our work well or poorly, and whether we will contact the neighbor who has just been told that her man was lost in a traffic accident or not.

Some situations are of such a nature that we cannot change them or wish them away. Sudden death is a scenario that Jaspers calls a boundary or limit situation. Other limit situations may be illness or experiencing various forms of loss such as losing your job, becoming divorced, going bankrupt, or being in a life-threatening situation. Jaspers believes death is the clearest limit situation, where we become separated from those we love and are attached to.

Common to all limit situations is that they lead to inner pain and suffering. These situations force us to realize that the world is unreliable. Pain and uncertainty challenge us to acknowledge our humanity. They remind us that we cannot take life for granted, that our whole existence is vulnerable, and that our life or the life of someone we love can be shorter than we had thought. Since human beings have self-awareness, we reflect on our own situations. The pain and suffering of limit situations throw us out of harmony, but asking questions related to our existence and the direction of our path can restore balance.

When suffering affects us, we become aware of both the boundaries in our own self and that we have limited ability to master and control the world around us. We simply know ourselves more powerfully than before. Such limit situations can also open us up to other people and to new perspectives, and we can be more aware of what is important in life and what responsibility we have to ourselves and to others. In this way, limit situations can mature us as human beings. While such existential turmoil feels negative, it also has a positive side, an aspect that is fresh and necessary, a visible sign of our human vitality. This distress of mind is an awakening that makes it clearer to us what is real and important in life and what is worth fighting for in times of suffering. Such struggles can encourage both moral and intellectual growth (Gatta 2015; Wikström 2001).

According to Norwegian theologian Lars Johan Danbolt (2002), the existential turmoil that becomes a weight to life in limit situations can lead to an inner work in two different ways. First, there is an explicit, visible, and clearly expressed work that others can see and understand. Second, a more implicit, hidden work is one that the person who experiences it is not always conscious of during the struggle (Danbolt 2002). The conscious and explicit work can be linked to grief work and reflections on experiences from life. It can be existential questions considered and worked on in relation to life and death, meaning, guilt and for-giveness, and responsibility. We try to figure out such questions of life by working with them both emotionally and cognitively in relation to our life-view.

The implicit, hidden work may be related to having children, getting older, going through various crises, or facing loss or death. The more invisible and silent processes are about being close to our own life-view and understanding the conditions under which we live. There is more to life than just understanding it. Some people never do quite discover answers to the big questions of life and death or their meaning. They can still feel that close proximity to other people, and nature can be of great help. According to Danbolt (2002), poetic language, more than everyday language, can be of particular help in the work on existential questions. In our life journey, we meet some wise people who help us under-stand what is happening in our deep inner places. One nursing student in charge of an elderly man we will call Sven, admitted to surgery for stomach cancer, told this story:

> It turned out that Sven had advanced cancer in the stomach that was spreading, so there was little that could be done for him. The doctor informed Sven about the situation after his operation. It was confusing to me because I saw no reaction from him after he had received this serious message. Had Sven understood the news? Did he dismiss the whole thing?
>
> Sven probably realized that I was confused because he was so calm, and one day he told me this: "I have been a captain on the Coastal steamer (which is a boat going with goods and people up and down the long Norwegian coast) all my adult life. Life has taught me that when it blows a storm, it is not possible to fight the wind. You just have to search for ways you can exploit the power of the wind and utilize it for your boat." Sven didn't say anything else, but I understood what he wanted to tell me: he understands what is happen-ing to him, but it is not his style to fight it or talk about it, so I do not need to know more.

In their summary article on spirituality, Weathers et al. (2016) show that spiritual care alleviates patients' suffering and enhances the experience of well-being. When patients are met spiritually, they are better able to adapt and master adversity and experience a sense of peace and inner strength. Other health-promoting findings related to spiritual care that were reported in these studies include an increased degree of hope, more motivation, and greater experiences of love and compassion and of knowing one's worth.

There were similar findings in a Norwegian study (Giske and Cone 2015), where nurses from various parts of healthcare were asked about why they looked at spiritual care as important for patients. The nurses said that they saw spirituality as part of life and being human, and therefore, part of nursing care. They saw that the spiritual was important for the patient to stay healthy and whole. Those who touched these struggles could see in their patients the pain in the questions they had, and the bittersweet feelings and guilt of patients who experienced darkening lives. Nurses were often surprised by the humor some patients could have in the face of death, the courage they showed, and the peace some patients had to hold on to when life was difficult.

At the same time, nurses and students noticed that with care of the spirit, patients were less depressed, emotional pain was diminished, anxiety was decreased, and patients found peace through conversations they identified as spiritual and existential. Nurses said that patients spoke about how the nurse could help them to stay strong and accept life the way it is, and that spirituality and peace affects patients living with chronic disease. It can also influence motivation and help them reach their goals and promote rehabilitation and healing (Giske and Cone 2015).

Reflection 1.10

- Have you experienced anything in your life that you could call a limit situation? Reflect on that.
- Do you recognize any of the pain and upset that Jaspers mentions?

- Think of patients you met. Have you been responsible for patients who experience limit situations? Have you seen any of the pain and distress they have experienced?
- Have you seen or heard expressions about how they work to resolve the challenges in their lives? How have they done this?
- What have you seen/heard/experienced that makes you recognize it as existential work?
- What do you think about the idea that spiritual care is an important part of nursing?

OUR PROFESSIONAL RESPONSIBILITY FOR SPIRITUAL CARE

Nursing's historical roots, ethical guidelines, common framework, theoretical frameworks, and documentation systems all evidence the fact that nursing care is based on a holistic human view and that spiritual care is a part of nursing's area of responsibility (ANA 2010). The *Code of Ethics* of the International Council of Nurses says: "Inherent in nursing is a respect for human rights, including cultural rights, the right to life and choice, to dignity and to be treated with respect" (ICN, 2021, p. 1). This includes what is valued, fit, and utilized in nursing practice. The American Nurses Association supports "nurses in providing consistently respectful, humane, and dignified care" (ANA 2015, "The Code"). Additionally, the ANA's policy statement for nursing underlines this as the professional responsibility of the nurse (ANA 2010). Moreover, part of the nurse's professional role is to maintain a commitment to society by serving with a "nonnegotiable ethical standard" (ANA 2015, "The Code"). Norway's professional nursing association also follows such ethical rules:

> *The nurse safeguards the individual patient's dignity and integrity, including the right to comprehensive nursing, the right to co-determination and the right not to be violated. . . The nurse supports the patient's hope, coping and life*

courage. . . The nurse takes care of the individual patient's need for comprehensive care.

(NSF 2012, p. 8)

Here we find the key words dignity, integrity, hope, coping, life courage, genuine caring, and wholehearted nursing, words that clearly show spiritual care is part of the nurse's responsibility. Regulations on the Norwegian common framework plan for health and social studies emphasize lifelong learning, something that is also important before spiritual care. After completing nursing education, the new graduate is required to have:

Knowledge of inclusion, gender equality and non-discrimination, regardless of gender, ethnicity, religion and beliefs, disability, sexual orientation, gender identity, gender expression and age, so that the candidate contributes to ensuring equal services for all groups in society.

(Forskrift 2017, p. 2.2)

The standards of care provide a framework for nursing care that patients should be able to expect. We are to offer equal services to patients regardless of race, color, gender identity, creed, religion, or beliefs. It can be challenging for students and nurses when we do not share beliefs or life-views with our patients.

The majority of nursing theories taught in nursing education are based on a view of the human being in which spiritual and existential issues are seen as part of being human and are the nurse's area of responsibility. We have chosen to present several nursing theories who have had and still have a great influence on modern nursing. American nurse scholar and teacher Virginia Henderson (1897–1996) was the first modern nurse who formulated what the nurse's distinctive function entails (McEwen and Wills 2017). Her nursing theory forms the basis of how the International Council of Nurses (*ICN*) formulated basic principles in nursing. Henderson said:

The nurse's outstanding function is to help man, whether sick or healthy, to perform the actions that contribute to health or recovery of health (or to a peaceful death), that this man would have done without help if he had the necessary strength, will and knowledge for this.

(Henderson 1978/1998, p. 45)

Henderson presents 14 basic areas where a person may need help from the nurse, of which one area is practicing their religion and acting as if the patient is right. Henderson was also the first to formulate the aim of nursing care includes to help a person to a peaceful death.

Two nurse theorists who include the spiritual in their theoretical models are Betty Neumann (Neuman 1996) with her NSM and Barbara Artinian (1991) with her AIM, who puts spirituality at the core of the human (McEwen and Wills 2017). Neuman believed that the person, or client, has the subparts of the "physiological, psychological, sociocultural, developmental, and spiritual, each of which is a subpart of all parts [that together]. . . forms the whole of the client" (Neuman and Fawcett 2002, p. 15). All these aspects of the person must be addressed by the nurse in order to promote stability of the system and work toward and/or maintain optimal wellness (McEwen and Wills 2017). Artinian puts the spiritual at the core of the person, both of the patient and the nurse, with spiritual, psychosocial, and biological subsystems that all need to be addressed when working toward a mutually negotiated plan of care (Artinian 1991). Additionally, "client spirituality and values are important in the assessment of client needs and within the resulting nursing process" (McEwen and Wills 2017, p. 155), so the nurse must address the deeply held beliefs and important practices that the patient values highly in order to provide whole person care.

The Norwegian nurse and philosopher Kari Martinsen (1943–present) is known around the world for her caring philosophy related to nursing care (McEwen and Wills 2017). Martinsen (2006) was inspired by the Danish theologian and philosopher, Knud Eilert Løgstrup (1905–1981), who wrote of the interactive relationship of the *one* and the *other*, a little like Martin Buber's *I and Thou* (Buber 1937/[1970]). Martinsen believes that nurses should be educated and trained so that they can consider and reflect on deeply important issues of their patient's fundamental human conditions, beliefs, and practices (Martinsen 2006). According to Martinsen, people are vulnerable and dependent on each other during illness., and our lives are borne up by the trust and compassion we have for each other (Kjær and Martinsen 2015). Martinsen's philosophy of care portrays three aspects of care. First, care is relational and human beings are dependent on each other. Second, care is practical, where one is actively and specifically involved in taking care of the other. And third, care is moral, with professional discernment and knowledge appearing in concrete actions (Martinsen 2006). Care is about learning how to handle power so that we care for the vulnerable. Such care leads to the courage and well-being of patients (Kjær and Martinsen 2015).

If we look at introductory books in the nursing profession, most have one or more chapters that deal with spiritual issues and spiritual care in nursing (Taylor et al. 2019a). Themes such as relief of suffering and strengthening of hope and life courage are presented along with a whole person perspective and the experience of context, hope, meaning, and/or transcendence (Haugan and Rannestad 2016; Taylor et al. 2019a). According to the nursing curricula from many countries globally, the right to exercise the view of life is a basic human need. This entails a more active responsibility for nurses to familiarize themselves with the life history of each individual patient and to facilitate the patient's need for care in the spiritual domain.

We believe that the life-view is part of the concept of health and whole person care and that being part of a faith fellowship or having a supported view of life can have a great impact on the quality of life and improve patient outcomes. By listening to the life story of those who can tell it themselves, or by compiling the life-view history by means of a leader or the family of those who cannot themselves convey it, the nurse can gain insight into what is important to the individual patient. The nurse can thus use the patient's life history and deeply important concerns to plan patient-centered holistic nursing care (Taylor et al. 2019a).

In nursing literature, healthcare professionals are responsible for assessing spiritual and existential needs. Such assessment can take place through the intake interview or in structured conversations during the course of treatment. It is important for health professionals to recognize expressions of spiritual needs or resources and to investigate what this means for the individual patient. We also emphasize the importance of explaining spiritual/existential care in the documentation system in a way that protects the patient's dignity and integrity, so that spiritual care is visible to those who work with the patient. Research shows that spiritual concerns and patients' needs for follow-up in this area of spirituality receive little space in the oral report at hospitals (Giske et al. 2018) and that there is insufficient documentation in the medical record system (Steenfeldt et al. 2018). Therefore, this is an area for growth in the healthcare system and among nurses.

Reflection 1.11

- To what extent has education given you the ability to act in whole person care?
- Do you have a nursing theory that you use in practice to help you think about nursing?
- Think of an example where you exercised spiritual care for a patient. What was that like for you?

SPIRITUAL CARE AS A DIFFICULT TOPIC

When it comes to spiritual issues, it seems to be a particular challenge in the Norwegian context, though this may also be true in other places where spirituality is considered extremely private. One study shows that Norwegian nursing students think it is more taboo for them to talk about faith, God, and spiritual things than it is to talk about sex (Giske and Cone 2012). Many Americans say that you should not talk about religion or politics, and with the divided society in the USA today, other issues such as racial discrimination, critical race theory, and white privilege are very "hot topics." The challenging thing is that we as nurses must be open to talk about whatever is important for the patient's healing path, regardless of the topic (Giske and Cone 2015; Taylor 2007).

One Norwegian study, which analyzed reflection notes from 385 first-year nursing students who had conducted a conversation with people about spiritual issues, showed that most students had never talked to anyone about such topics before (Kuven and Giske 2019). The theme they were supposed to talk about was what gives hope and meaning in life, whether the person had a faith tradition or not, and what was important in relation to the patient's need (Stoll 1979). The students were encouraged to talk to a person who had an illness experience, and one of the questions was whether this experience led to changes in their own beliefs and/or faith. The analysis showed that the conversation challenged the students to become better acquainted with themselves and who/what gave them hope or pain in their own life, as well as to reflect on what they themselves believed. The students recognized that the study requirement was difficult and that the questions were very private, so they dreaded it. The conversations challenged them to go beyond their own comfort zone in order to complete the required assignment. Reflection notes showed that the vast majority of students were pleasantly surprised by what came out in the conversation, and that those who already knew the person they conversed with discovered that the conversation helped them become more familiar at a deeper level (Kuven and Giske 2019).

Nurses also say that there can be little tolerance for a cultural taboo about addressing religious and spiritual questions in clinical practice (Cone and Giske 2013b; Giske and Cone 2015; McSherry and Jamieson 2013; Ødbehr et al. 2015). Both in acute care and in psychiatry, nurses communicate that they feel they must be very cautious in this area because it is so personal and private to talk about spiritual issues (Cone and Giske 2017; Medås et al. 2017). This is a challenge for those of us who work with nursing education, for students, for healthcare providers, and for the individual nurse (Molzan and Sheilds 2008; Taylor 2007). Nurses have a professional responsibility to ensure that we develop so that we can focus on patients and their families in such a way that what is important to the patient can come to light. Moreover, nurses are accountable to align our expertise with professional standards that include the spiritual domain, and not to just passively practice values that the society around us claims (ANA 2015).

> **Reflection 1.12**
>
> • What do you think about whether or not it is taboo to talk about spiritual needs and resources for patients in nursing?
>
> • Is there a difference in the way various wards, units, or departments address a patient's spiritual needs or concerns? If so, what is this difference about?

ONE LEARNING SPIRAL IN THREE PHASES

Spiritual care practice can be facilitated by utilizing a learning spiral that emerged from our research among nursing students (Giske and Cone 2012) and teachers (Cone and Giske 2013b; Cone and Giske 2013a). This spiral of learning can improve the nurse's ability to recognize and follow-up patients in the spiritual domain and to look at it as part of holistic nursing. Open Journey Learning Spiral has three phases of a learning journey that provide the structure for the three middle chapters of this handbook (see Figure 1.1). Since nurses are on a lifelong journey in our profession, these phases repeat with every new patient and each new thing that we learn.

Phase one, which we present in Chapter 2, deals with how students and nurses can prepare personally and professionally for patient connections (Giske and Cone 2012). This is done by

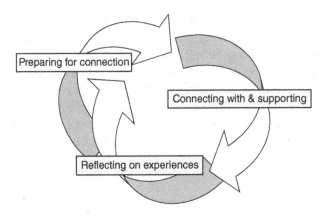

FIGURE 1.1   Open Journey Learning Spiral (Based on Cone and Giske 2013a).

becoming more familiar with themselves and by gaining knowledge of different approaches to spiritual care that we provide along the way. Students can use this collection of resources related to spirituality and spiritual care to help them grow and become more aware of the spiritual domain.

Chapter 3 discusses phase two, which involves connecting with and building relationships with patients (Cone 1997; Taylor 2007). Students learn to recognize cues and follow up on spiritual issues that are important to the patient. Each patient must be met at a deep level and be supported along his or her healing path. Both needs and resources that the patient has are addressed in order for nurses to help patients toward the best health and quality of life possible.

The third phase of the learning spiral is presented in Chapter 4, namely the importance of reflecting on experiences from practice, both alone and together with others, in order to develop competence for spiritual care. Written reflections, such as journaling on spiritual encounters, are important to inner growth. Some students and nurses experience that it can be challenging to create a professional relationship with patients and keep rapport intact when spiritual conditions occur (Giske and Cone 2012; Ødbehr et al. 2015).

Finally, we end our handbook with a discussion in Chapter 5 of the need to be lifelong learners and to grow both personally and professionally in our spiritual care competence (Van Leeuwen and Cusveller 2004). We remind students and nurses to practice self-care in practical ways in order to thrive in the nursing profession and to work toward creating a healing environment wherever you serve. We hope that this handbook will serve as a practical guide for increasing the capacity of nurses to provide patient-centered whole person care.

REFERENCES

Aadnanes, P.M. (2012). *Livssyn* [Lifeviews], 4e. Universitetsforlaget. [Norwegian language book but a synopsis can be found in Bråten and Everington, 2018.]

Alligood, M.R. (ed.) (2018). *Nursing Theorists and their Work*, 9ee. Mosby Elsevier.

American Nurses Association [ANA] (2010). Nursing's social policy statement: The essence of the profession. https://www.nursingworld.org/practice-policy/nursing--excellence (accessed 22 March 2022).

American Nurses Association [ANA] (2015). *Code of ethics for nursing.* https://www.nursingworld.org/practice-policy/nursing-excellence/ethics/code-of-ethics-for-nurses (accessed 22 March 2022).

Artinian, B. (1991). The development of the intersystem model. *Journal of Advanced Nursing* 16 (2): 194–205. https://doi.org/10.1111/j.1365-2648.1991.tb01625.x.

Artinian, B., Conger, M., and West, K. (2011). *The Artinian Intersystem Model.* Springer.

Best, M., Butow, P., and Oliver, I. (2015). Do patients want to talk to their doctor about spirituality? A systematic literature review. *Patient Counseling and Education* 98 (11): 1320–1328. https://doi.org/10.1016/j.pec.2015.04.017.

Bråten, O.M.H. and Everington, J. (2018). Issues in the integration of religious education and worldviews education in an intercultural context. *Intercultural Education* 30 (3): 289–305. https://doi.org/10.1080/14675986.2018.1539307.

Buber, M. (1937)/[1970]. *I and Thou*. [Tran. from German by W. Kaufman]. Simon & Schuster.

Carson, V.B. (2011). What is the essence of spiritual care? *Journal of Christian Nursing* 28 (3): 173.

Chan, M.F., Chung, L.Y.F., Lee, A.S. et al. (2006). Investigating spiritual care perceptions and practice patterns in Hong Kong nurses: results of a cluster analysis. *Nurse Education Today* 26 (2): 139–150.

Clark, J. (2013). *Spiritual Care in Everyday Nursing Practice: A New Approach*. Palgrave Macmillan.

Cone, P. (1997). Connecting: The experience of giving spiritual care. In: *The Intersystem Model: Integrating Theory and Practice* (ed. B.M. Artinian and M. Conger), 270–288. Sage.

Cone, P.H. (2020). Facilitating spiritual care for whole person patient-centered care. *Online Journal of Complementary and Alternative Medicine* 1 (2): 1–2. https://doi.org/10.33552/OJCAM.2019.01.000507.

Cone, P.H. and Giske, T. (2013a). Open journey theory: intersection of journeying with students and opening up to learning spiritual care. *Journal of Nursing Education and Practice* 3 (11): 1–9.

Cone, P.H. and Giske, T. (2013b). Teaching spiritual care: a grounded theory study among undergraduate nursing educators. *Journal of Clinical Nursing* 22 (13–14): 1951–1960. https://doi.org/10.1111/j.1365-2702.2012.04203.x.

Cone, P.H. and Giske, T. (2017). Nurses' comfort level with spiritual assessment: a mixed method study among nurses working in diverse healthcare settings. *Journal of Clinical Nursing* 26 (19–20): 3125–3136. https://doi.org/10.1111/jocn.13660.

Danbolt, L.J. (2002). *Den underlige uka: de sørgende og begravelsesriten* [The strange week: the mourners and the funeral rite]. Verbum Forlag.

Edwards, H., Speight, J., Bridgman, H., and Skinner, T.C. (2016). The pregnancy journey for women with type 1 diabetes: a qualitative model from contemplation to motherhood. *Practical Diabetes* 33 (6): 194–201.

Fowler, M. (2020). Evangelism in patient care: an ethical analysis. *Journal of Christian Nursing* 36 (3): 172–177. https://doi.org/10.1097/CNJ.0000000000000622.

Fowler, M., Kirkham, S.R., Sawatzky, R., and Taylor, E.J. (2011). *Religion, Religious Ethics, and Nursing*. Springer Publishing.

Forskrift om felles rammeplan for helse- og sosialfagutdanninger (2017). https://lovdata.no/dokument/SF/forskrift/2017-09-06-1353

Frankl, V. (1946/1959). *Man's Search for Meaning. [Translated from German into English by Ilse Lasch]*. Beacon Press.

Gatta, G. (2015). Suffering and the making of politics: perspectives from jaspers and Camus. *Contemporary Political Theory* 14 (4): 335–354.

Giske, T. (2010). Sårbarheit, makt og tillit: tillit – den gode bru mellom sårbarheit og makt, eksemplifisert med pasientar innlagde på sjukehus til utgreiing [vulnerability, power and trust: trust – the good bridge between vulnerability and power examplified by patients hospitalized for diagnostic workups]. *Michael* 2: 252–259.

Giske, T. and Cone, P.H. (2012). Opening up for learning: a grounded theory study of nursing student education on spiritual care. *Journal of Clinical Nursing* 21 (13–14): 2006–2015.

Giske, T. and Cone, P.H. (2015). Discerning the healing path: how nurses assist patients spiritually in diverse healthcare settings. *Journal of Clinical Nursing* 24: 10–20. https://doi.org/10.1111/jocn.12907.

Giske, T., Melås, S.N., and Einarsen, K.A. (2018). The art of oral handover: a participant observational study by undergraduate students in a hospital setting. *Journal of Clinical Nursing* 27 (5–6): e767–e775. https://doi.org/10.1111/jocn.14177.

Great Norwegian Encyclopedia [Store norske leksikon]. (2017). Livsyn [Lifeview]. https://snl.no/livssyn (accessed 22 March 2022).

Haugan, G. and Rannestad, T. (2016). *Helsefremming i spesialisthelsetjenesten* [Health promotion in the specialist health services]. Damm Cappelen.

Henderson, V. (1978). *The Principles and Practice of Nursing*. Macmillan. [Trans. 1998 by Oslo University Press *Sykepleiens natur. Refleksjoner etter 25 år*. Universitetsforlaget].

Herdman, T.H. and Kamitsuru, S. (ed.) (2017). *Nursing Diagnoses 2018–2020: Definitions and Classification*, 11ee. Thieme.

Horsfjord, V. (2017). *Religion I Praksis [Religion in Practice]*. Universitetsforlaget.

International Council of Nursing [ICN]. (2021). *ICN Code of Ethics for Nurses*. Author. https://www.icn.ch/system/files/2021-10/ICN_Code-of-Ethics_EN_Web_0.pdf.

Kjær, T.A. and Martinsen, K. (2015). *Utenfor tellekantene. Essay om rom og rommelighet.* [Outside the counting edges. Essay on space and spaciousness]. Fagbokforlaget.

Krauss, J.C., Warner, J.L., Maddux, S.E. et al. (2016). Data sharing to support the cancer journey in the digital era. *Journal of Oncology Practice* 12 (3): 201–208.

Kristofferson, N.J., Nortvedt, F., Skaug, E-A., and Grimsbø, G.H. (2016). *Grunnleggende sykepleie 1: Sykepleie – fag og funksjon* [Fundamentals in nursing 1: Nursing – the discipline and role function]. Glydendal Akademisk.

Kuven, B.M. and Bjørvatn, L. (2015). Spiritual care: part of nursing? *Christian Nurse International* 5: 4–8.

Kuven, B. and Giske, T. (2019). Talking about spiritual matters: first years nursing students' experiences of an assignment on spiritual care conversation. *Nurse Education Today* 75: 53–57. doi: 10.1016/j.nedt.2019.01.012.

Leenderts, T.A. (2014). *Person og profesjon. Om menneskesyn og livsverdier i offentlig omsorg* [Person and profession: About view of man and life values in healthcare]. Gyldendal Akademiske.

Martinsen, K. (2006). *Care and Vulnerability* [Originally in Norwegian: English translation by L.E. Kjerland]. Akribe.

McEwen, M. and Wills, E.M. (2017). *Theoretical Frameworks for Nursing*, 5ee. Lippincott Williams & Wilkens.

McSherry, W. and Jamieson, S. (2013). The qualitative findings from an online survey investigating nurses' perception of spirituality and spiritual care. *Journal of Clinical Nursing* 22: 3170–3182.

McSherry, W. and Ross, L. (2010). *Spiritual Assessment in Healthcare Practice*. M & K Publishing.

Medås, K.M., Blystad, A., and Giske, T. (2017). Åndelighet i psykisk helseomsorg: et sammensatt og vanskelig tema [spirituality in mental healthcare: a complex and difficult topic]. *Nordisk Tidsskrift for Sygepleje* 31 (4): 273–286. https://doi.org/10.18261/issn.1903-2285-2017-04-04.

Minton, M.E., Isaacson, M.J., Varilek, B.M. et al. (2018). A willingness to go there: nurses and spiritual care. *Journal of Clinical Nursing* 27 (1–2): 173–181. https://doi.org/10.1111/jocn.13867.

Molzan, A.E. and Sheilds, L. (2008). Why is it so hard to talk about spirituality? *The Canadian Nurse* 104 (1): 25–29.

National Health Service [NHS] for Scotland (2009). *Spiritual Care Matters: An Introductory Resource for all NHS Scotland Staff.* Edinburgh: National Education Service.

Neuman, B. (1996). The Neuman systems model in research and practice. *Nursing Science Quarterly* 9 (2): 67–70. https://doi.org/10.1177/089431849600900207.

Neuman, B. and Fawcett, J. (2002). *The Neuman Systems Model,* 4ee. Prentice Hall.

Nolan, S., Saltmarsh, P., and Leget, C. (2011). Spiritual care: working towards an EAPC task force. *European Journal of Palliative Care* 18: 86–89.

Norsk Sykepleierforbund [NSF]. (2012). Yrkesetiske retningslinjer for sykepleiere [Professional ethics guidelines for nurses]. In: *ICNs etiske regler [International Council for Nursing Code of Ethics].*

North American Nursing Diagnosis Association [NANDA]. (2016). Nursing diagnoses. http://www.nandanursingdiagnosislist.org (accessed 22 March 2022).

Norwegian Ministry of Health and Care Services [NMHC]. (2009). *Opptrappingsplan for psykisk helse 1999–2006.* [Step-up plan for mental health services 1999–2006], p. 6.

Ødbehr, L.S., Kvigne, K., Hauge, S., and Danbolt, L.J. (2015). A qualitative study of nurses' attitudes towards' and accommodations of patients' expressions of religiosity and faith in dementia care. *Journal of Advanced Nursing* 71 (2): 359–369.

Pargament, K. (2007). *Spiritually Integrated Psychotherapy: Understanding and Addressing the Sacred.* The Guilford Press.

Petiprin, A. (2016). Neuman's Systems Model. *Nursing Theory.* https://nursing-theory.org/theories-and-models/neuman-systems-model.php (accessed 22 March 2022).

Pew Research Center [PRC] (2021). PRC statistics on religion in the United States. https://www.pewforum.org/2015/11/03/u-s-public-becoming-less-religious (accessed 22 March 2022).

Royal College of Nursing [RCN] (2011). *Spirituality in Nursing: A Pocket Guide.* London: Royal College of Nursing.

Rykkje, L. (2016). Forståelse av åndelighet og åndelig omsorg for gamle mennesker – en hermeneutisk studie [Understanding spirituality and spiritual care for the elderly: A hermaneutic study]. *Nordisk Tidsskrift for Helseforskning* 12 (1): https://doi.org/10.7557/14.3780.

Rykkje, L.R., Eriksson, K., and Råholm, M.B. (2013). Spirituality and caring in old age and the significance of religion: a hermeneutical study from Norway. *Scandinavian Journal of Caring Sciences* 27: 275–284. https://doi.org/10.1111/j.1471-6712.2012.01028.x.

Statistics Norway. (2019). Statistisk Sentralbyrå [Culture and faith = Religion and lifeview]. http://www.ssb.no/kultur-og-fritid?de=Religion+og+livssyn (accessed 1 November 2021).

Steenfeldt, V.Ø, Sommer, C., and Wiggers, M.V. (2018). Trialog. *Fag og Forskning* 3: 14–37.

Stoll, R.I. (1979). Guidelines for spiritual assessment. *American Journal of Nursing* 79 (9): 1572–1577.

Taylor, E.J. (2007). *What Do I Say? Talking with Patients about Spirituality.* Templeton Foundation Press.

Taylor, E.J. (2012). *Religion: A Clinical Guide for Nurses.* Springer Publishing.

Taylor, C.R., Lynn, P.B., and Bartlett, J.L. (2019a). *Fundamentals of Nursing: The Art and Science of Patient-Centered Care*, 9ee. Wolters Kluwer.

Taylor, E.J., Gober-Park, C., Schoonover-Shoffner, K. et al. (2019b). Spiritual care at the bedside: are we practicing what we preach? *Journal of Christian Nursing* 36 (4): 238–243.

Torskenæs, K.B., Kalfoss, M.H., and Sæteren, B. (2015). Meaning given to spirituality, religiousness and personal beliefs: explored by a sample of a Norwegian population. *Journal of Clinical Nursing* 24 (23–24): 3355–3364.

Van Leeuwen, R. and Cusveller, B. (2004). Nursing competencies for spiritual care. *Journal of Advanced Nursing* 48 (3): 234–245. https://doi.org/10.1111/j.1365-2648.2004.03192.x.

Watson, J. (1997). The theory of human caring: retrospective and prospective. *Nursing Science Quarterly* 10 (1): 49–52. https://doi.org/10.1177/089431849701000114.

Watson, J. (1999). *Human Science and Human Care: A Theory of Nursing*. Jones & Bartlett.

Weathers, E., McCarthy, G., and Coffey, A. (2016). Concept analysis of spirituality: an evolutionary approach. *Nursing Forum* 51 (2): 79–96. https://doi.org/10.1111/nuf.12128.

Wei, H. and Watson, J. (2011). Healthcare interprofessional team members' perspectives on human caring: a directed content analysis study. *International Journal of Nursing Sciences* 6 (1): 17–23. https://doi.org/10.1016/j.ijnss.2018.12.001.

WHO-QoL SRPB Group (2006). A cross-cultural study of spirituality, religion, and personal beliefs as components of quality of life. *Social Science and Medicine* 62 (6): 1486–1497.

Wikström, O. (2001). *Den outgrundliga människan [The Unfathomable Man]*. Borås: Nature & Culture.

CHAPTER 2

Preparing for Spiritual Care

The first step to preparing for spiritual care is to know oneself on a deeper level. This includes having good knowledge in areas such as communication, ethics, culture, religion, and deeply held beliefs about illness and treatment. In this handbook, there is no room to go into detail on each of these areas, but we will emphasize the importance of seeing the process of spiritual care in context, and we will refer to good resources that address such details. In this chapter, we will look at different ways that we can improve ourselves in order to meet patients and their relatives in the best possible way in the spiritual arena. This is a lifelong learning process because no human or situation is exactly alike; we all have similarities and differences, and we grow and change throughout life.

We begin by going into different aspects of knowing ourselves at a deeper level and of identifying the things and people that influenced our personal history and life-view. We discuss why this is important in the exercise of spiritual care. To that end, we invite readers into various activities that can help in the process of

The Nurse's Handbook of Spiritual Care, First Edition. Pamela Cone and Tove Giske.
© 2022 John Wiley & Sons Ltd. Published 2022 by John Wiley & Sons Ltd.

becoming better acquainted with ourselves. Later, we examine our values and beliefs with a view to becoming more comfortable with who we are, not trying to change these elements. Finally, we look more closely at general and special expertise that we need before we can practice or facilitate spiritual care.

KNOWING YOURSELF AND YOUR OWN HISTORY

A *life story* is the story of the individual's journey through life; it tells about our life and the people and situations that have influenced us (Harrison 2009). Here, the big and small are woven together for a story about who I am and what has been and is important in my life. Our life story is told more or less consciously, in light of the culture, time, and beliefs we have. *Life story* is an approach that expresses identity and self-understanding of a person. Whoever has a reflected relationship with a personal life history has markers to understand her/his own thoughts and feelings in the face of others' life stories.

Life story applies to me; it is my *ego story* or *I-story*. It has a start, a middle, and it has an end; it has time and space, experiences, cities and places, people, books, music, and much more that are important in my life and my history (Harrison 2009). When we tell our *I-story*, we like to emphasize different parts of it in relation to what processes we are in and who we tell it to. It will also change as we mature and gain new life experiences. In some individuals, a pattern may develop in which one places greater emphasis on the positives that have happened in life, while others may have an ego history where negative and painful experiences have the most space.

As human beings, we live together with others, so my life story will always be related to other people. We are fluttering into their lives and living in other stories, and they are doing the same with us. Together, we become we-tales. We all have such *we-stories*. The family, neighbors, friends, classmates, work colleagues, patients, and relatives we meet are the human beings who are woven together in my *I-story* to become *we-stories*. Our identity does not grow simply out of the *I-story*, it is also tied to the larger story we are a part of, what was there before us, and what follows after we are gone.

Universal stories or *all-stories* are stories that anyone can tell and that apply to all human beings (Harrison 2009). There are many such parallel all-stories, and all cultures have their all-stories. All-history in our culture has many elements in it. In Norway, for example, the Norse shaped Norwegian culture in the Viking Age, where men were very courageous and traveled far and women were strong and independent and responsible for home affairs. In the eleventh century, the spread of Christianity and the Christian faith and values of western society largely shaped the values of Norway today. Many implicit values are held across the Norwegian culture whether or not an individual has a personal faith. The legacy of antiquity has also seen its traces in the form of art, governance, sports, and architecture. Adventures, myths, literature, philosophy, and history are other elements that weave into our great all-story.

In the United States, Americans have the universal history of fighting for our freedom to choose our own way of life, beliefs, and practices, which is, perhaps, one reason that the issue of slavery of the black people in America and subsequent racial discrimination and injustice is such an anathema to many of us. Americans fought for our freedom, and then we enslaved other people! We took away the freedom of black people from them, and then we had to fight another war within our nation for their emancipation and to make sure that all people are part of our American values of "everyone is created equal" and "all have equal rights and freedoms." Going against our original core beliefs by embracing slavery of people from Africa set our nation up for racial discrimination and injustice that is part of the all-story of America today, but especially among black Americans.

We are born into all-history, into our country and family history before we even have our own story. In this way, no one creates her or his identity from scratch; we become part of something bigger before we can understand and tell our own I-story. The all-story is about giving an overview, and it helps us to understand the I- and we-stories in a larger context. Being part of the same all-story provides a deep sense of community and a backdrop of understanding that is often silent to us (Harrison 2009). Meeting with others who tell their I-story, say from another all-story story than mine, can help me get rid of all that I take for granted so that I can share with others without bias. For example, the African American community has an all-story about the heritage of slavery and cruelty their ancestors experienced that people who did not grow up within that group often fail to understand. This lack of understanding is true of many cultures where there has been tragedy, generalized suffering, or extreme injustice. It is not right to say there are no differences, that differences do not matter, or that we are all the same since we are equal, because differences actually do matter, and we must acknowledge them and learn to listen to the all-story or we-story of others. We meet more and more people in the healthcare system today who have an all-tale that is different from the African American one or the Norwegian one, and each one is important to those who are from that particular group. If the social beliefs, norms, and values as well as rules of behavior are different from what we are familiar with, we need to gain knowledge and to take time for conversation and active listening in order to understand others more fully.

Human beings tell their single stories of small and large events in life as we try to organize our history into wholeness. The all-telling can help with such an orientation and can put life and experience into a larger context, especially when we experience limit situations that bring us up against some sort of wall or border. All history, however, is open and forces no one to adapt. As we grow older as human beings, a process of individualization takes place, and the individual can tell his/her life more or less consciously in or out of the all-history into which one is born. This is true of African Americans today as the USA struggles to come to grips with our nation's past and how it has negatively influenced our present society and social norms. In America, each of us needs to recognize where we have gotten out of sync with our original, faith-based beliefs and practices, or the non-faith based deeply held beliefs some have, and take ownership of the stereotypes, prejudices, and injustices that are so prevalent across America.

In the secularized and individualistic society of many nations today, the evidence of intolerance with differences is more and more frequent. Secularization and pluralization have meant that the all-telling in Norway is not as clear-cut as it was earlier. Norwegian psychiatrist Gordon Johnsen (1905–1983) said that what we are conscious of we can do something with, but what we are not conscious of does something with us. This means that anyone who has a reflected relationship to self and to the I-history, we-history, and all-history that speaks into their life knows what they stand for and can more easily be open and clear in the face of others who have differences (Harrison 2009). According to Victor Frankl, "Between stimulus and response there is a space. In that space is our power to choose our response. In that response lies our growth and our freedom" (Jones 2016, para. 1 #15). We continue to work at opening up our minds in this chapter.

Reflection 2.1

- How does this I-story relate to me?
- Who/what are important people and events in this story?
- What we-stories do you talk about? Does this change from childhood, to adolescence, and to the age of accountability or understanding?
- What parts of the all-history are important for you to pass on to your children?

BACKGROUND AND CONTEXT MATTER

In a Norwegian study of how nursing students learn to exercise spiritual care, it emerged that the students' background, including world view, knowledge, and earlier experiences, influence their level of maturity (Giske and Cone 2012). This is true of both strengths and weaknesses in the face of patients with difficult health conditions or spiritual concerns. The students experienced a particular challenge when meeting patients who had another belief/life-view or other values than themselves (Giske and Cone 2012).

A later study with Norwegian nurses who recognized and followed up patients spiritually showed that the nurse's personal identity and background together with education and age had significant influence on how they exercised their nursing care (Giske and Cone 2015). Individual maturity, developing through personal and professional experience, can help the nurse know him/herself at a deeper level and thus help us dare to open up to what is important to the patient. In other words, we can say that our upbringing, our own I- and we-history, our personal and professional experiences, and the knowledge and understanding we gain characterize who we are as a person, and thus who we are as a nurse and the nursing care that we perform (Baldacchino 2011; Giske and Cone 2015; Van Leeuwen et al. 2008).

The nurse's outlook on life and willingness to provide spiritual care have been shown to be closely tied to the nurse's experience of having a good role model or with a precedent they experienced as having met patients spiritually (Cone and Giske 2017; McSherry and Jamieson 2013; Ødbehr et al. 2015). Thus, these nurses usually see spiritual care as important for their nursing care. People being comfortable with their own spirituality also seems to influence the nurse's view and experience of the professional responsibility for spiritual care. In Chapter 1 we explained that providing spiritual care is about relationship, meaning, and transcendence (Weathers et al. 2016), which is more than beliefs, rituals and practices, or religion. Spiritual concerns outside the nurse's "comfort zone," or the nurse being uncomfortable with the spiritual domain (Minton et al. 2018) is described as what makes it difficult to talk to others about spiritual/existential conditions (Cone and Giske 2017; Giske and Cone 2012).

The most important single factor when it comes to whether or not nurses themselves provide spiritual care is therefore the self-awareness of the nurse. Self-awareness can be defined as a multi-dimensional, introspective process in which one is continuously aware of and examines and understands personal thoughts, feelings, beliefs, and values. We can use this reflection process when we want to act "in a conscious and authentic way" (Eckroth-Bucher 2010, p. 304). Vietnamese Buddhist monk Thich Nhat

Hanh is a globally known Zen master who believed that the practice of mindfulness helps us to get in touch with ourselves and others in a meaningful way: "With mindfulness, you can establish yourself in the present in order to touch the wonders of life that are available in that moment." He said that "The most precious gift we can offer others is our presence" (Jones 2016, para. 1 #12). Self-awareness is existence-oriented and presence-oriented and can help us to be truly engaged and fully present with others.

Reflection 2.2

The Royal College of Nursing (RCN 2011) has a pocket- sized pamphlet with some good questions to help you think through and assess your own spirituality:

- Do you have a way you work to find meaning with what happens to you?
- What sources of support and help do you have when your life is difficult?
- Would you like to have someone who could help you?
- Would you like to have someone who could help you think or talk through health problems or life habits you have?

KNOWING YOURSELF AT A DEEPER LEVEL

Students, teachers, and nurses talk about the spiritual as something that is deep and personal, something that has to do with the whole of life's attitudes and actions (Rykkje et al. 2021). It is about what we hold to as true and most important, as we understand ourselves in the big context, and it can accommodate doubts and uncertainties we have in relation to the big questions in life. The spiritual care provider is like an anchor that helps provide meaning and clarity in life by being there for and with the patient in their healing process (Cone and Giske 2013b; Giske and Cone 2012, 2015). Thus, it is important to understand the spiritual side of us that integrates all aspects of our person so that we can face life's challenges knowing what we believe and reach out to others, whether they believe as we do or not (Cone 2016; Nielsen 1984)

These thoughts underline the crucial importance of knowing ourselves and being consciously aware of our own beliefs and values. Working with such questions is part of living fully as a human being. Knowing our own vulnerability, life pain, and doubts can be difficult, but it can help us to new power and strength to move forward in life. Sharing stories from one's own life or practice through the writing of reflections can be a good way to learn from each other, often in reflection together. Reading biographical material can also help expand our understanding and give us the courage to stand firm in challenging processes. Here is a small story about knowing life pain and having to think again about what is important and meaningful to people.

> *Kari is 19 years old and goes to a doctor for a checkup before she has to move to the city to start her nursing program. The doctor's checkup reveals ovarian cancer, and further studies show that the cancer is aggressive in nature. The doctor tells Kari and her family that he recommends removing both ovaries and follow up with chemotherapy; otherwise, there is small chance that she will survive. Kari is signed up for surgery immediately after getting the first word of this cancer diagnosis. She has not had time to think, but the healthcare team is certain that her only chance is to act quickly. Her family agrees; however, without ovaries, it will not be possible to conceive and bear a child, which Kari has longed for since she was a little girl.*

Reflection 2.3

- What would be your first reaction if you were this young woman?
- How would you feel about this diagnosis and proposed surgery?

- What would you choose if you were in this situation?
- What would you say and do if you were the nurse caring for this young woman?

Our understanding of the greater context of life is not static; it changes as we live, learn, and experience life's challenges. Our beliefs and values therefore become increasingly conscious, coherent, and integrated into our lives as we process them. This applies to both patients and healthcare professionals. Both patients and students/nurses can work on such issues, especially in periods where life is more challenging, such as in Kari's situation in the story above (Rykkje et al. 2021). Our experiences are interwoven with the spirit and work together with our view of life and the doubts or concerns we can recognize and how we interpret our lives. This is done in many ways, from integrating the simple and everyday life events to the big connections where we do not have sure knowledge or experience to build on, but such mental and emotional work is demanding and takes time. At this point, we risk the threat of "standing alone, naked and vulnerable; then there is nothing for anyone to rely on other than hope and promise" (Brager and Wisløff 1990, p. 20), and it takes great courage to stay in the learning and growing process to move toward maturity (Giske and Cone 2015).

EXERCISES TO GET BETTER ACQUAINTED WITH YOURSELF

In this section, we invite you to do various activities that can help you become better acquainted with yourself on a deeper level. These exercises can be used individually, in groups, in classes, or during a clinical post-conference session at the hospital.

DRAWING YOUR LIFE TREE

This task is to draw your life as a tree. Here you are invited to work in a creative way where the tree of life is used as a metaphor for discovering new aspects of yourself. For equipment, you need a clear sheet of paper and colored pens, pencils, or crayons. When you proceed with this activity, set aside 15–20 minutes. You need peace and a willingness to open yourself up. If you do this together with others, place yourself so that you have some room around you (if possible) and set yourself up in a bit of isolation, cut off from the others around you.

Box 2.1   Are You Ready to See Yourself as a Tree?

1. Draw your roots. What have you celebrated in life and still find nourishing? What do the roots of your tree look like? Where do they go; what is their source of nourishment?

2. You are the tree trunk, and you have branches that are life activities and relationships. How does your tree stand (solid, firm, weak, bent)? How have you grown? What is the pattern of your branches?

3. Does the tree have any fruit? What fruit have you borne?

4. During this work, pay attention to your inner dialogue.

This exercise is *not* about being good at drawing. Drawing and colors are chosen to promote a symbolic expression for the person you are and the people who have been and are important in your life. If you feel barriers to drawing, use your non-dominant hand – the one you draw the worst with. When you do the task, do not think too much; just give yourself over to the process, and your thoughts will come in a flow where you know how to express yourself, and what colors and shapes you are going to use to make your life tree.

Reflection 2.4

When you have drawn your life tree drawn, think about what you have drawn.

- What people and situations have been important in your life – positive and negative?
- How has this shaped you into who you are today?

By putting words onto what is expressed in the drawing and the inner dialogue you had along the way, you will be able to understand more deeply and become more aware of the person you are and the processes you are in right now. If you have done this task in a group, call two or three together to discuss your experience. In the conversation, just share what you want; do not feel obligated to share it all. If you carry out the exercise alone, write down the discoveries and your thoughts; be as detailed as you can so that you can reflect again as you read over what you wrote.

Reflection 2.5

- What are your wishes/desires for the future?
- What resources do you have in you and around you that can make it possible for you to reach what you want?
- What challenges do you have that do or may make it difficult for you?
- Is there anyone you can invite into your processes so that you can reach your wishes/dreams?

WORKING WITH YOUR OWN VIEW OF LIFE AND PERSONAL STORY

This task is an invitation to be better acquainted with our philosophy of life as well as what has been involved in influencing this. The assignments are inspired by the work of educator, journalist, and developer Jens-Petter Jørgensen (2014). He has extensive experience in working with life-view narratives in groups. Writing and sharing a life history provides an opportunity for what professionally is called narrative life interpretation, which means using stories to work with one's own identity and gaining a deeper understanding of how we understand and interpret our own lives. This exercise can be done in depth or more superficially.

We recommend that you work with one or more others who are interested in working with their own vision of life. You can either meet several times and ask one question about the activity each time, or you can choose to work with all the questions at one time. The time needed depends on how many meet and how many questions are raised. Before you start work, talk about the fact that discussion with the others in the group is voluntary and other people's confidentiality must be maintained. Think about whether you need to anonymize the information you share and talk about the fact that what is shared in the group is tacit-silence and not to be shared with others.

Everyone will need pen and paper and enough room for to sit and write individually and then sit together in a circle and share what you each have written down. Clarify how long you will spend on individual writing and how much time each individual gets to share in the group. We recommend that you spend 10–15 minutes writing down your thoughts first. The conversation in the group can be organized so that the individual gets 6–7 minutes to share what they have written. By "just" listening attentively to what the others are saying, we open ourselves up to understanding and wondering, and we accept what the other gives. After one has listened to a story, the rest of the group can give feedback on how each person experienced hearing the story and what each one found particularly touching. Do not discuss *what* was told because that type of discussion opens the group up for counter-arguments and critical comments, something that can hamper the sharing of personal stories about how the individual experiences his/her life.

Box 2.2   Activity for Working Out Your Own Life-View

Here are suggestions for topics for writing and conversation:

1. What characterizes the environment where you grew up, in relation to your view of life?

2. What was your childhood home like? What relationship did you have with mother and father? What view of life did they have? Are there others in your family (siblings? extended family?) who have been important to you in the development of your view of life?

3. Have you had important role models for your view of life? Who were these and why were they important to you?

4. If you have a faith, how did you come to that faith? If you do not have a faith, what is your life-view?

5. What kind of image do you have of God today? If you do not have any faith belief, do you have a picture of the God you do not believe in? Has this changed over the years? Is there any connection between your image of God and your self-image?

6. What space do you give to personal experiences and crises that influenced the development of your philosophy or view of life?

7. What longings and expectations do you have for your view of life in the years that lie ahead? What do you want to be true for you in five years? What are you longing for? What can you do to make these dreams come true?

BECOMING AWARE OF VALUES IN YOUR OWN LIFE

This exercise is about giving yourself time to think about values and being more certain of what it is most important in your life. The exercise will also invite you to know and reflect on what it means to have values and to lose values. For supplies, you need a sheet of paper and pen or pencil. When you proceed with this task, first set aside 10-15 minutes to quiet your thoughts. You need peace and willingness to open yourself up. If you do this together with others, place yourself so that you have some room around you (if possible), focus within yourself, and cut out the others around you. Think about what you actually think spiritual care is. It is easy to reduce it to faith, religion, and beliefs. This is part of it, but it matters that we delimit and broaden it.

In this exercise, we will clarify the important values for us. Values are expressed in the ideals and beliefs we have about what is right and wrong. Values include what is most important to us, what gives our life meaning, and what is worth striving for. This shows up in relationships and norms for how we should act and behave toward others. Values can also be characteristics we have held highly as being what we rely on. These can include a great working capacity, being able to listen, showing empathy, and being able to set limits. Values can be concrete things like the value of having money, house, car, dress, and creating or achieving a project or a dream.

In Chapter 1, we referred to the European Association of Palliative Care (Nolan et al. 2011); they refer to spirituality where one dimension relates to value-based assessment and attitudes and what is important in relationships with patients. Moreover, we showed how the American Nurses Association's professional role statement (ANA 2010) as well as the *Code of Ethics for Nurses* (ANA 2015) maintain that it is the nurse's responsibility to create an environment in which patients and relatives feel that their own values are respected. When you do the next activity, do not think too much; rather, pay attention to how it feels for you to do this exercise and what your inner dialogue is.

By putting words to what you experienced in this exercise and the inner dialogue you had along the way, you will be able to understand and become more aware of who you are, what is most important to you, and the life processes you are in. If you have done this task in a group, call two and two together. In the conversation, you share just what you want, not everything. If you carry out the exercise alone, write down the discoveries and your thoughts about the whole process.

Box 2.3   Activity for Values Clarification

Start this way:

1. Write down five relationships or beliefs that are most valuable to you.

2. It doesn't need to be the five most valuable things in your life; the most important thing is that you can say that what you write down is a value for you. Don't think too much; just write down what comes to your mind.

3. Look at the five values you wrote down. Many of the patients we encounter experience limit situations and are in life situations where they have lost functions, relationships, freedom, security, and/or perhaps time due to illness. These are important losses where they may not have been able to make a choice; life is like that. In this exercise, you can choose what is valuable to you.

4. Give a simple name to any values you have identified; describe each one.

5. Pay attention to your inner dialogue when you are doing this and notice how it feels for you to do this. Again, listen to your inner dialogue.

6. Delete one value. What is least important to you? Do this again until you find identify the two most important values.

7. Finally, clarify and define these two values. You do not need to prioritize between them or choose which one is the most important.

Reflection 2.6

- What was it like to delete any of your initial values?
- How did your inner dialogue affect you during this task?

- What do you think it means when we, as nurses, create an environment in which patients and relatives feel that their values are respected?
- How can you use insights from this exercise to meet patients and relatives?

According to the Artinian Intersystem Model, evaluating the knowledge, values/attitudes, and actions/behaviors of both the nurse and the patient in order to develop a mutually negotiated plan of care (Artinian et al. 2011) is of primary importance. By knowing ourselves more deeply, we can be better prepared to assist our patients with thinking through and processing new information. If they need more knowledge, we can provide it or gather it for them. If they need to understand something to see if it aligns with their deeply held values, we can help them clarify that by listening and being a sounding board. Finally, if they are struggling with how to manage a challenging diagnosis, or with some choice or behavioral issue, we can problem solve with them to come up with a good plan. However, our ability to do that with the patient is dependent on our own self-understanding and openness as well as our courage and willingness to stay in difficult situations where we may not have answers or we feel differently than the patient. We must accept and support the patient by listening and asking good questions.

THE ART OF ASKING GOOD QUESTIONS

Practicing to become aware of the difference between asking open or closed questions is important in nursing. Try a couple of situations at home or among friends to ask open questions (those that do not have yes/no answers) and listen to what the person tells you. Notice how the content of the conversation and the relationship develops. Then try to use closed questions where the other can answer yes or no and see if the conversation changes.

Reflection 2.7

- Think about how you talk to people in different situations.
- You have different relationships with friends, family, children, parents, colleagues, patients, and relatives during one day. Think about how you interact with them.
- What kind of questions do you use – open or closed questions? Think about what makes you choose the question types you do.

Noticing how patients talk can help us to understand where they are in their process and thus justify our action when we take the conversation further. The Norwegian nursing researcher Venke Ueland (2002) says that the language of suffering or spiritual/existential thought is often a hesitant and searching language. Some patients have never talked about this before and may need nurses who are sensitive and patient in the art of listening. So notice if the patient speaks in full sentences, is confident and precise with a good flow, or if the person is hesitant, thinks a lot, searches for words, has sentences that are not completed, and if the conversation comes to a halt.

American nurse researcher Elizabeth Johnston Taylor (2007) encourages nurses to use attentive engaging and active listening skills in order to figure out what, if anything, they should say to their patients. Much about knowing the person relates to the content they are talking about as well as how they are expressing it. Note whether the person is using everyday language or whether they use spiritual vocabulary and religious words and expressions (Cone 2016). These things can tell us a lot about a person and what information they may want or need. Does the patient use metaphors when he or she speaks? Listening to whether the person speaks most about facts or most about feelings provides important information to us about what the patient is concerned about and whether or not they try to process and cope with their situation (Giske and Artinian 2008). As we gain experience through conversations with different patients, we will be able to use the information about how patients talk and what they are talking about to help us ask good and important questions in our nurse-patient conversations.

TWO SIMPLE QUESTIONS

Building a good and trusting relationship with the patient provides the best foundation for being able to converse about spiritual health/existential concerns. Furthermore, it is a good way to prepare to think through various questions that may be appropriate for assessing patients, both on admission and along the way. British nursing researchers Linda Ross and Wilf McSherry have introduced two questions that they call 2Q-SAM, which stands for 2 Questions-Spiritual/Holistic Assessment Model (Ross and McSherry 2018). These two questions are: *What is the most important thing for you now? How can we help*? These two simple and open questions can help the nurse exercise patient-centered care because patients have the opportunity to say what is important to them here and now.

If we ask a patient in the morning, the answer to be judged may be that the patient is tired because he had no sleep. This can invite a further question about why no sleep. If one asks the patient later in the day, the patient can answer that he needs a wheelchair because of a man who plans to visit. The nurse then understands that they can help by getting the wheelchair to the patient. Ross and McSherry (2018) tell a story where the patient, by having the wheelchair, is able to reach a quiet place in the canteen where he can talk to his husband about how to have his funeral since he knows he is going to die soon. The wheelchair is thus one way of giving the patient both physical and spiritual care, but it first makes the nurse address a practical need that leads later to addressing a deep concern of the patient.

By asking this simple question: *What is the most important thing for you now?* The nurse opens the door for patients to come up with what lies on their heart. Often, however, it takes a little more time and testing to ensure that what the patient has at heart will come forward. By listening to what the patient says and the way he says it, we can sense if we need to ask one more time: *Is there anything more important to you now?* By listening and showing interest, such a simple question can open up for the patient to realize that this student/nurse is interested in what is at stake in my life. By asking the question a third time: *And is it more important for you right now?* the patient can understand that this student/nurse is really interested in me. When it is clear what is most important to the patient, we can ask: *How can I help you?* This also is an open question that puts us in the learner mode with the patient teaching us or explaining to us what they need most, whether it is to address a concern or to help them access their own resources. Then we can plan follow-up care from there.

Reflection 2.8

- Do you have experience in asking patients a question similar to: What is the most important thing for you now?
- Can you imagine trying out the question: What is the most important thing for you now? And how can I help you? Ask this of a couple of friends and see what experience you have.
- Prepare yourself to ask the first question in your next patient encounter.

QUESTION GUIDES FOR SPIRITUAL CARE

There are many examples of slightly more detailed data collection guides (McSherry and Ross 2010) for research and for use in practice. We have chosen to present three different data collection guides that are often used and that can be of help and inspiration. These are short, with main points that are easy to think about, and questions can be tailored to different situations and patients. We recommend, before you apply one or more of these in practice, you work on understanding the main areas of the individual guide and practice them with others. When you know the data collection guide well, you can more easily customize the questions according to what you consider fit in the meeting with the individual patient. As you gain experience, you will probably create your own questions that you have seen work to open up conversations about spiritual conditions for the patient group you are working on.

The first question guide, developed by the American nursing researcher Ruth Stoll (1979), is one of the earliest data collection guides for spiritual care published. Stoll indicates four main areas related to faith tradition, what gives hope and strength, how spirituality is related to health, and one's view of life, all of which are important to address. Her first question addresses what thoughts the person has about God. Since we perceive this as a very personal question in many countries and cultures, we recommend that you place this question at the end and start with the broad and open questions before going to the specific. Begin with the question on the patient's basis for hope and strength. Examples of sub-questions are under each main area.

Box 2.4   Spiritual Care Assessment by Stoll

1. *Basis for hope and strength*
   - Who do you turn to when you need help? Is this/are these available to you?
   - In what way do they help you?
   - What basis do you have for hope and strength?

2. *The relationship between spirituality and health*
   - What thoughts do you have in relation to becoming ill, being ill, or being in this particular situation?
   - What do you think will happen ahead related to your health situation?
   - Is there any special concern for you? Or something you're particularly worried about?

3. *View of life and philosophy of life*
   - What and/or who do you believe in?
   - Do you feel that your belief system helps you? If yes: Do you want to tell me how?
   - Has this situation led to any changes in your daily rituals or practices?

The next part of this question works for those with an acknowl-
edged religious belief:
  • What books and/or symbols are helpful to you?
  • Is there any religious practice that is important to you?
  • Has this situation led to any changes in relation to your
    religious practices?

4. *Concept of God or the Transcendent*
  • Is God or deity or the sacred important to you?
  • If no, end this line of questioning. If yes: Can you
    tell me how?
  • Does prayer help you? What happens when you ask?
  • How do you describe God? What/Who do you worship?

US physician Christina Puchalski (2013) developed **FICA**,
the second data collection guide we provide. FICA is an acronym
for **F**aith, **I**mportance, **C**ommunity, and **A**ddress. More detailed
information is listed on her homepage on the development of the
data collection guide, as well as other resources in relation to
spiritual care (http://smhs.gwu.edu/gwish/clinical/fica).
Here are questions for the four areas in the FICA disseminate data
collection guide:

Box 2.5   FICA Spirituality Assessment by Puchalski

1. *Faith, truth and belief:*
  • Do you consider yourself to be spiritual or religious?
  • Is it important for you?
  • Do you have spiritual strategies that help you cope with
    stress/troubling times?
  • If the patient says no, you can ask this question that
    is relevant to all patients: What does your life mean?

(Continued)

Box 2.5   (Continued)

2. *Important issues:*
   - What significance does this belief have in your life?
   - Does it have any spiritual significance in how you care for yourself and your health?
   - How does it affect the spiritual decisions you make regarding health?

3. *Communities:*
   - Are you part of a spiritual or religious community? Communities can be such things as a church, temple, mosque, or a likeminded group, a family or yoga group, etc. A group or community can be a strong support system for patients.
   - Do you have a group that you love or that is important to you and supports you?

4. *Address relevance to the care:*
   - How do you want us to follow this up in further planning together with you?
   - How can we help you now?

HOPE, the last data collection guide we present, was developed by American scholars Gowori Anandarajah and Ellen Hight (Anandarajah and Hight 2001) in order to integrate the spiritual into data collection and treatment of patients. HOPE stands for **H**ope, **O**rganized religion, **P**ersonal spirituality and practice, and **E**ffects. The four areas include suggested questions the health worker can ask.

Box 2.6 HOPE Spiritual Assessment by Anandaraja and Hight

1. *Hope: Basis for hope, purpose, strength, peace, love, and affinity*
   - What basis do you have for hope, strength, comfort, and peace?
   - What do you hold onto in difficult times?
   - For some people, religious or spiritual truth is a source of hardship or strength to deal with ups-and-downs in life. How is this working for you? Has this changed over time for you?

2. *Organized religion*
   - Do you consider yourself part of an organized religion?
   - What parts of religion are useful and/or less useful to you?
   - Are you part of a religious or spiritual community?
   - What is most important to you?

3. *Personal Spirituality and Practice*
   - Do you have a personal spirituality, regardless of organized religion? What is it?
   - Do you believe in God?
   - If so, what kind of relationship do you have with God?
   - What parts of your spiritual practice are most useful to you personally (e.g. prayer, meditation, reading texts, music, walking, communicating with nature)?

4. *The Effect on medical treatment and challenges at the end of life*
   - Does being ill affect the ability to do the things that usually help you in the spirit area or does it affect your relationship with God?

(Continued)

Box 2.6   (Continued)

- As a doctor/nurse, is there anything I can do to help you access the resources that usually help you?
- Are you concerned about any conflicts between you and the medical situation you are in or the follow-up nursing care or decisions you need to make?
- Would it be helpful for you to talk to the priest or another spiritual leader?
- Are there any particular conditions or restrictions I should be familiar with regarding the medical treatment (e.g. diet or use of blood product)?
- If the patient is very ill: What do you think of the treatment you will receive the next days/weeks/months?

These assessment guides or tools can be practiced with each other or with friends and then with patients until they form a sound base for your patient assessments. The tools do not need to be strictly followed, with every question answered. The nurse must go at the pace set by the patient (Giske and Cone 2015) and allow the patient to lead in the discussion with the nurse simply providing prompts that elicit more dialogue and help the patient to express what is on his or her mind and heart, what is deeply important to him/her.

Reflection 2.9

- Which one of these three data guides did you like best? What are your arguments for that?
- Do you have experience using some of the questions suggested here? What is your personal experience with these types of questions?

- If you have no experience with asking such questions of patients, is there one of these question guides that you would like to try out?

We conclude this section with some questions from the Spiritual Care Nursing Guide developed by the Royal College of Nursing (2011) in the UK. In the same way that we consider the physical needs of our patients, it is important that we also consider the patients' deeply personal distressing concerns and/or strengths and resources from the outset. As we can see, the questions that the RCN suggests are similar to the three data collection guides shown above.

Box 2.7   RCN Assessment Guide for Spiritual Assessment

1. What basis for help and support do you have when life is difficult?
2. Do you have a way to help you find meaning in what is happening to you?
3. Do you want to talk to someone who can help you think through your situation?

PREPARING FOR THE "I-DON'T-KNOW-WHAT-TO-DO" SITUATIONS

Through the study of students (Giske and Cone 2012) an interesting expression emerged: "I-don't-know-what-to-do" situations. Such situations come to us all sooner or later, situations when we get confused, where we do not know what to say or do. Is it possible to pre-empt such situations?

Yes, it is. We must first be self-aware and know our own thoughts, feelings, and expectations of ourselves and our patients. By thinking through times when we feel a sense of confusion or discomfort, we will learn to stop a second and think about what is happening in the moment. It is possible to decide ahead of time that when we come into a challenging situation, we will rather be courageous at such times than leave the situation and possibly neglect a patient concern. Looking at the patient's face or a relative's face can help us to understand what is going on inside the patient. The eyes and the face of the patient will often show us whether they want us to go on or not, and whether we will be rejected if we do proceed. Having thought through such situations beforehand and having decided to stand in the uncertainty gives us a readiness to face I-don't-know-what-I-should-do situations.

Reflection 2.10

- Have you experienced such I-don't-know-what-to-do situations? If you have, go through the situation in your mind and reflect on what happened and how you experienced the situation.

- How do you talk to yourself when you are in professional situations where you do not know what to do?

- How can you prepare for the next I-don't-know-what-to-do situation?

- What is most challenging for you in such situations?

One very important thing to remember is that you do not need to have the answer to everything. Patients do not expect us to know everything, but nurses often expect that of ourselves. So, when we do not know what to say or do, then we may lose our courage to pursue a deep patient concern. Most patients simply want genuine compassion and engagement and active listening so that they can process their deeply important issues with us as a sounding board.

WHAT SIGNAL DO YOU SEND OUT?

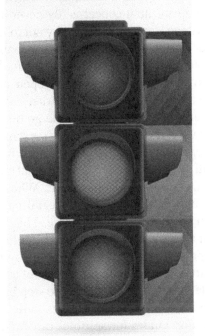

In the first part of this chapter, we focused on the importance of knowing ourselves. Moreover, we have looked at how we can ask questions so that spiritual and existential concerns can come forward.

Before we finally look at what skills are needed for spiritual care, we will borrow an idea that the Danish nurse Grete Schärfe presented in 1988 to emphasize that patients read the students and nurses, their words and expressions, and interpret them in relation to how or if we are open to understanding the significance of spiritual issues. Schärfe (Schärfe 1988; Schärfe and Rosenkvist 2008) uses the image of a traffic light. If a nurse sends out a red light, they signal: "Stop, do not take it up with me, I am not interested." This can be done by ignoring what the patient expresses, downplaying or dismissing it as unimportant. Red light can also express itself by the nurse being too busy.

The yellow light signals a pending hold where it is up to the patient to take up spiritual concerns. By never asking questions about faith, existence, or spirituality or by not following this up in an interview or during the stay, the entire responsibility is transferred to the patient. This can be challenging for the patient who is already feeling vulnerable. By using open and non-specific questions such as 2Q-SAM mentioned earlier, a yellow light nurse can gently determine if he or she should go on or if the patient really does not want the nurse to address personal issues.

A nurse sends a green light to patients when listening and asking in-depth questions about conditions that are about spiritual challenges and/or well-being of patients. When words that are about tragedy and existence are an integral part of the nurse's language, such themes naturally emerge. This can be done, for example, by making eye contact while listening, by physically touching the patient's shoulder or hand, or by mentioning the beauty of nature, informing the patient about a religious activity that is available, offering to ask a priest to stop by if they wish, or by using more general questions such as those we have written about in "Question guides for spiritual care." The green light is seen and understood intuitively by most patients through the attitude and actions of the nurse that express kindness, openness, tolerance, respect, and empathy (Cone and Giske 2021).

The traffic light image illustrates that we ask with a basic approach in the face of patients who can open up or close down about what is important to them. As we saw in Chapter 1, spiritual care is an integral part of whole person or holistic nursing that we are responsible for assessing and following up in the same way as the physical part of nursing care. It indicates that nurses should signal green light as the main response to spiritual concerns. The fact that a student or nurse expresses a green light for spiritual care does not mean that topics in conversations with all patients will include the spiritual. Being a professional means that it is the patient's situation that determines whether it is important or not to pursue spiritual/existential concerns and that we are open and clear when it matters to the patient.

In practice, sometimes patients send out trial signals to check whether the student or nurse understands what they are absorbed in or experiencing. If we do not understand, both the patient and the nurse will come away from the situation without being challenged to resolve a deep issue. Sample signals from patients will be easier for nurses with a green light attitude to capture than for those with a red light, to use Schärfe's metaphor. To illustrate this from a patient perspective, we have an excerpt of an interview with a young woman we will call Lisa who has experienced many hospitalizations. Lisa has reflected a lot over how she can identify the nurse who tolerates deep concerns, and how to communicate to the nurse, especially on those bad days:

Interviewer:	Help me to understand how you read nurse attitudes.
Lisa:	I have been admitted many times, both in intensive and here at intermediate care, but they addressed only my asthma. They don't ask me about really important things to me, it seems they are afraid of it. If they see me crying, then they will avoid asking. I have trained my whole life to seem happy, so I can show that, but sometimes I get overwhelmed. Because I see that it stresses them, I try not to show it.
Interviewer:	How do you see what a nurse tolerates?
Lisa:	Well, I see that they are uncomfortable, nervous and such, fluttering the eyelids and uneasy in the body. Some get very quiet; they don't know what to say. I see that they are uncertain. Others say they have to go do other things. But others are not afraid to come to me, I see it in the eyes of the soul, they are not afraid. I feel safe when they are there. Some people touch me

Interviewer: gently on my shoulder, because it is good that they are close and have time when we talk about the existential, that they are not 15 feet from my bed – then I do not feel that we have contact.

Interviewer: Please tell me more about this.

Lisa: I feel that many are uncomfortable. Not that they do not want to help me, but they do not have education so that they are able to talk to people about how they have deep feelings, they lack experience and feel helpless. They need education so they are prepared and can understand how they should respond when patients tell their stories. They should try to find something nice to say, because it is OK to feel that you can feel it with the patient. Accept what is; don't worry if a patient is sad, because if you do worry, the patient will try to hide it from you.

Reflection 2.11

- What "light" do you signal to your patients when it comes to spiritual care? How aware are you of the attitude that you project to your patients?
- If your light is not green, what is behind this choice?
- If it varies, what is it that affects this variation in your attitude?

GENERAL AND SPECIAL COMPETENCE IN SPIRITUAL CARE

What skills do you need for spiritual care? As we have seen, the nursing care plan should be from a whole person, patient-centered view, and the nurse should seek to create an environment in which the human rights of the individual, family, and society are respected no matter their values, norms, and beliefs (ANA 2015; ICN 2021). The general spiritual care competence that patients and society should be able to expect all nurses to have is about being able to identify patients' spiritual needs and resources, and be able to evaluate them and plan how they should follow up (see the BSN Standard for Spiritual Care Competencies developed by the EPICC Network of Spiritual Care Scholars on http:// blogs.staffs.ac.uk/epicc/). It is interesting that research on nurse training in spiritual care reveals that such care not only influences the nurse's personal and professional growth, but their patients have many positive effects and outcomes that enhance recovery (Vasblom et al. 2011). Being able to listen, support, and encourage patients as well as to put practical matters into action is expected of all nurses in providing patient-centered, whole person care.

Moreover, all nurses should be able to talk with patients about how they can best follow up and whether it is necessary to refer to others on the interdisciplinary team. It is not a defeat to refer the patient to the hospital priest/chaplain or a local priest, pastor, imam, deacon, or other person the patient would like to speak to about deeply personal and important concerns. This general competency consists of having a caring meeting with patients (RCN 2011; Van Leeuwen and Cusveller 2004; Van Leeuwen et al. 2008), where the nurse considers and follows up on spiritual conditions in the same way as physical and psychosocial conditions in a patient.

A connection happens between the nurse and patient as trust and rapport are developed. As shown in Figure 2.1, nurses need to start with acceptance of patients' deep concerns, whether their own beliefs, values, and view of life are similar to or different from the patient. Nurses need to listen and learn about the patient, support and engage with the patient, and be fully present in the moment with that patient while being aware of self in order to keep building the rapport that can facilitate spiritual care.

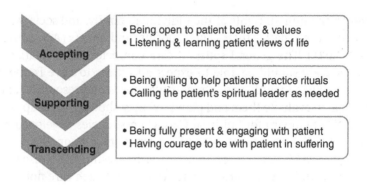

FIGURE 2.1 Connecting: a basic social process of spiritual care (Cone 1997).

It is important to know the limits of your own competence and know when the time is right to pull in others. In spiritual assessments, it is important to be aware that the nurse must not destroy the trust shown by the patient by referring the patient further before understanding what the patient needs. Unfortunately, patients may be referred to "philosophy of life specialists" because the nurse feels uncertain or unsafe in such conversations. If the patient wants a person who can listen to his/her thoughts and trusts that the student/nurse is able to stay and listen, a referral to another professional may seem or feel like a rejection. As we travel this learning journey in our personal and professional lives, it is important to remember these oft-quoted words attributed to French American Quaker activist, philanthropist, and reformer Stephen Grellet (1773–1855): "I expect to pass through this world but once. Any good therefore that I can do or any kindness that I can show to any fellow creature, let me do it now. Let me not defer or neglect it, for I shall not pass this way again" (Seebohm 2016, p. 18).

Special competence in spiritual care is related to the student and the nurse as a person and is about personal threats, challenges, and experiences one has had in life as well as formal and informal knowledge, education, and training that the individual has beyond what the nursing education provides (Leenderts 2014).

One European pilot study conducted in four countries (Ross et al. 2016) and a large longitudinal study of 21 universities in eight European countries (Ross and McSherry 2018) both showed that students say that understanding personal spirituality and spiritual care were the two most important conditions that affect the students' self-reported ability to exercise spiritual care.

Having a reflected relationship with one's own view of life makes it possible for us to meet patients who share our view of life in a deeper way than those who do not share the same view of life. Being an atheist, agnostic, or humanist gives the student or nurse special insight, experience, and knowledge in this perspective that gives him/her a special expertise for patients with those life-views. This special insight is also true when having a faith tradition that is shared by the patient. Furthermore, life experiences can provide a student/nurse with personal expertise that comes in addition to education of various types. Losing a child, going through a serious illness, or having relatives who are seriously ill and/or dying are life experiences that give special expertise. When students/nurses meet patients and relatives in similar situations, they will be able to understand these situations in a different way than those who do not have such experiences.

Further education and/or special interests that enable one to read and acquire knowledge and insight beyond personal experience will also provide special expertise. For those who have not been provided with the BSN Standard for Spiritual Care Competencies, it would be a good idea to go to the free EPICC Network website (http://blogs.staffs.ac.uk/epicc/) and learn more about competencies on their own. This personal competence enables the nurse to confirm existential and spiritual conditions and to go deeper into conversations with patients than one can expect from a nurse who does not have such an experience in his/her background. In order for this special expertise not to be simply a "cop out" with us depending on other team members or to create the impression that spiritual care is just for those who are especially interested, it is important that there are conversations among the team members. There needs to be an openness in the colleague community and work environment, where anyone in the working community can talk about various beliefs, experiences, and knowledge and interests of individual employees. In this way, patients will also be able to have access to the expertise found among the personnel working in their unit or ward.

> **Reflection 2.12**
>
> • Consider your own general expertise. What are your strengths, and what do you need to develop further?
> • Put words on what is your special competence. How can you add to the community you are part of? How do/can you use your special competence with patients and their unique needs?

In Chapter 3, we move on from preparing for a nurse–patient encounter to actually connecting with the patient. The better prepared we are, the more able we will be to engage with the patient and make a trustful connection. In the first author's initial spiritual care study, the most important factor in nurses and students actually providing spiritual care was found to be their own comfort with personal spirituality (Cone 1997). As we said earlier, this is a lifelong process, so start where you are and keep working on honestly knowing yourself and becoming more comfortable with who you are and what you believe. Your spiritual journey is one of the most important gifts you can give your patients as you care more and more effectively for their inner spirits.

REFERENCES

American Nurses Association [ANA] (2010). *Nursing's Social Policy Statement: The Essence of the Profession.* https://www.nursingworld.org/practice-policy/nursing-excellence (accessed 22 March 2022).

American Nurses Association [ANA] (2015). *Code of Ethics for Nursing.* https://www.nursingworld.org/practice-policy/

nursing-excellence/ethics/code-of-ethics-for-nurses (accessed 22 March 2022).

Anandarajah, G. and Hight, E. (2001). Spirituality and medical practice: using the HOPE questions as a practical tool for spiritual assessment. *American Family Physician* 63 (1): 81–89. https://www.aafp.org/afp/2001/0101/p81.html (accessed 21 July 2021).

Artinian, B., Conger, M., and West, K. (2011). *The Artinian Intersystem Model*. Springer.

Baldacchino, D.R. (2011). Teaching on spiritual care: the perceived impact on qualified nurses. *Nurse Education in Practice* 11: 47–53.

Brager, E. and Wisløff, D.S. (1990). *Så lenge vi lever. Bruksbok for helsearbeidere i møte med åndelige behov* [As long as we live: Handbook for health workers in meeting spiritual needs]. Cappelens Forlag.

Cone, P. (1997). Connecting: a basic social process of spiritual care. In: *The Intersystem Model*, 1ee (ed. B. Artinian and M. Conger). Sage.

Cone, P.H. (2016). Commentary on the importance of spiritual literacy. *Christian Nurses International: Partnerships (A Journal of NCFI)* 1 (7): 17–19.

Cone, P.H. and Giske, T. (2013b). Teaching spiritual care: a grounded theory study among undergrad nursing educators. *Journal of Clinical Nursing* 22 (13–14): 1951–1960.

Cone, P.H. and Giske, T. (2017). Nurses' comfort level with spiritual assessment: a mixed method study among nurses working in diverse healthcare settings. *Journal of Clinical Nursing* 26 (19–20): 3125–3136. https://doi.org/10.1111/jocn.13660.

Cone, P.H., & Giske, T. (2021). Hospitalized patients' perspective on spiritual assessment: A mixed-method study. *Journal of Holistic Nursing* 39 (2): 187–198. doi: 10.1177/0898010120965333.

Eckroth-Bucher, M. (2010). Self-awareness. A review and analysis of a basic nursing concept. *Advances in Nursing* 33 (4): 297–309.

EPICC Network. (2021). Spiritual care educational Standard & Spiritual care self-assessment tool. Retrieved from http://blogs.staffs.ac.uk/epicc/.

Giske, T. and Artinian, B. (2008). Patterns of "balancing between hope and despair" in the diagnostic phase. A grounded theory study of patients at a gastric ward. *Journal of Advanced Nursing* 62 (1): 22–31.

Giske, T. and Cone, P.H. (2012). Opening up to learning: a grounded theory study of nursing student education on spiritual care. *Journal of Clinical Nursing* 21 (13–14): 2006–2015.

Giske, T. and Cone, P.H. (2015). Discerning the healing path: how nurses assist patients spiritually in diverse healthcare settings. *Journal of Clinical Nursing* 24: 10–20. https://doi.org/10.1111/jocn.12907.

Harrison, B. (Ed.) (2009). *Life story research* [4 volume work]. Sage. https://uk.sagepub.com/sites/default/files/upm-binaries/24510_Final_Ch_Prelims_Vol_I.pdf (accessed 22 March 2022).

International Council of Nursing [ICN]. (2021). *ICN Code of Ethics for Nurses*. https://www.icn.ch/system/files/2021-10/ICN_Code-of-Ethics_EN_Web_0.pdf (accessed 22 March 2022).

Jones, M. (2016). INC: 28 Incredibly motivating quotes to start your week. https://www.inc.com/matthew-jones/28-motivating-mindfulness-quotes.html (accessed 3 December 2021).

Jørgensen, J-P. (2014). *Når troen setter spor. Hjelp til å arbeide med din troshistorie* [When faith leaves traces: Help in working on your faith history]. Luther Forlag.

Leenderts, T.A. (2014). *Person og profesjon. Om menneskesyn og livsverdier i offentlig omsorg* [Person and profession: About view of man and life values in healthcare]. Gyldendal Akademiske.

McSherry, W. and Jamieson, S. (2013). The qualitative findings from an online survey investigating nurses' perception of spirituality and spiritual care. *Journal of Clinical Nursing* 22: 3170–3182.

McSherry, W. and Ross, L. (2010). *Spiritual Assessment in Healthcare Practice*. M&K Pub.

Minton, M.E., Isaacson, M.J., Varilek, B.M. et al. (2018). A willingness to go there: nurses and spiritual care. *Journal of Clinical Nursing* 27 (1–2): 173–181. https://doi.org/10.1111/jocn.13867.

Nielsen, E.A. (1984). *Menneske – medmenneske – Den åndelige omsorg i sykepleien* [Man – Fellow human being – Spiritual care in nursing]. Universitetsforlaget.

Nolan, S., Saltmarsh, P., and Leget, C. (2011). Spiritual care in palliative care: working towards an EAPC task force. *European Journal of Palliative Care* 18: 86–89.

Ødbehr, L.S., Kvigne, K., Hauge, S., and Danbolt, L.J. (2015). A qualitative study of nurses' attitudes towards' and accommodations of patients' expressions of religiosity and faith in dementia care. *Journal of Advanced Nursing* 71 (2): 359–369.

Puchalski, C.M. (2013). Integrating spirituality into patient care: an essential element of person-centered care. *Polskie Archiwum Medycyny Wewnętrznej* 123 (9): 491–496.

Ross, L. and McSherry, W. (2018). The power of two simple questions: The nurses who devised a spiritual care model for acute settings explain how it works and why it can save you time as well as enhancing your person-centred practice. *Nursing Standard* 33 (9): 78. https://doi.org/10.7748/ns.33.9.78.s22.

Ross, L., Giske, T., Van Leeuwen, R. et al. (2016). Factors contributing to student nurses'/midwives' perceived competence in spiritual care: findings from a European pilot study. *Nurse Education Today* 36: 445–451. https://doi.org/10.1016/j.nedt.2015.10.005.

Royal College of Nursing [RCN]. (2011). *Spirituality in Nursing: A Pocket Guide.* London: Royal College of Nursing. https://docplayer.net/16388491-Spirituality-in-nursing-care-a-pocket-guide.html (accessed March 2022).

Rykkje, L., Søvik, M.B., Ross, L. et al. (2021). Enhancing spiritual care in nursing and healthcare: a scoping review to identify useful educational strategies. *Journal of Clinical Nursing.* https://doi.org/10.1111/jocn.16067.

Schärfe, G. (1988). *Spiritual Care: The Role of the Nurse? A Literature Review.* Copenhagen: Danish Nurses' Council.

Schärfe, G. and Rosenkvist, S. (2008). Bliv parat til åndelig omsorg [Be prepared for spiritual care]. *Sygeplejersken [The Nurse]* 8: 44.

Seebohm, B. (2016). *The Memoirs of the Life and Gospel Labors of Stephen Grellet*, 1e/1860, 10e/2016. Wentworth Press.

Stoll, R.I. (1979). Guidelines for spiritual assessment. *The American Journal of Nursing* 79 (9): 1574–1577.

Taylor, E.J. (2007). *What Do I Say? Talking With Patients About Spirituality*. Templeton Press.

Ueland, V. (2002). Sykepleieren og den åndelige/eksistensielle samtalen. Hvordan kan vi konkret samtale med pasienten? [the nurse and the spiritual/existential conversation. How can we concretely talk with the patient?]. *Kreftsykepleie [Cancer Nursing]* 3: 11–19.

Van Leeuwen, R. and Cusveller, B. (2004). Nursing competencies for spiritual care. *Journal of Advanced Nursing* 48 (3): 234–245. https://doi.org/10.1111/j.1365-2648.2004.03192.x.

Van Leeuwen, R., Tiesinga, L.J., Middel, B. et al. (2008). The effectiveness of an educational programme for nursing students on developing competence in the provision of spiritual care. *Journal of Clinical Nursing* 17 (20): 2768–2781. https://doi.org/10.1111/j.1365-2702.2008.02366.x.

Vasblom, J.P., van der Steen, J.T., Knol, D.K., and Jochemsen, H. (2011). Effects of a spiritual care training for nurses. *Nurse Education Today* 31: 790–796. https://doi.org/10.1016/j.nedt.2010.11.010.

Weathers, E., McCarthy, G., and Coffey, A. (2016). Concept analysis of spirituality: an evolutionary approach. *Nursing Forum* 51 (2): 79–96. https://doi.org/10.1111/nuf.12128.

CHAPTER 3

Connecting: Recognizing and Following up Spiritual Encounters

In Chapter 2, we looked at how students and nurses can prepare so that we develop a reflective relationship with our own values and life experiences. This is important because it is about shaping each of us into a nurse who is prepared for deeply personal encounters with patients. In this chapter, we discuss how we can connect with patients, build rapport, and identify and address issues that are in the spiritual domain. Nurses and other healthcare professionals often say that they do not know how to identify something as spiritual, when to address it if they recognize an intangible issue that is important to the patient, and what to say or do when there is something within the inner spirit of their patients (Koenig 2013). Therefore, we talk about how we can concretely recognize, evaluate, and follow up on spiritual issues, including existential, religious, relational, and philosophical

The Nurse's Handbook of Spiritual Care, First Edition. Pamela Cone and Tove Giske.
© 2022 John Wiley & Sons Ltd. Published 2022 by John Wiley & Sons Ltd.

conditions, concerns, and resources of patients in the same way as we consider and follow up on their physiological and psychosocial needs. We also look at how we can document the spiritual care that we provide. The chapter concludes with a review of various factors that affect the spiritual care process.

THE IMPORTANCE OF RAPPORT BUILDING

In her nursing theory on developing the nurse-patient relationship, American nurse and teacher Joyce Travelbee (1926–1973) took the positivist human view that characterized the nursing profession in the 1960s (Travelbee 1971). Travelbee was primarily inspired by the writings of three scholars: Danish theologian and existentialist Søren Kierkegaard (1813–1855), American existential psychologist Rollo May (1909–1994), who wrote *Man's Search for Himself* (1953), and Jewish psychiatrist and Holocaust survivor Victor Frankl (1905–1997), who wrote *Man's Search for Meaning* in 1946 (Alligood 2018). All of them addressed the deep inner searching that human beings go through when they experience vulnerability and suffering, and they recognized and wrote about the relational nature of humankind.

According to Travelbee, nursing is an interpersonal process in which the nurse should, if needed, help the person, family, or community to find out what the experience of illness and suffering leads to and how to deal with it (Alligood 2018). Coping with stress, feeling vulnerable, and balancing hope versus despair are patient concerns that nurses should address through active listening, effective communication, and using themselves therapeutically, all key factors in her nursing theory (Travelbee 1971). In order to accomplish their service to patients, nurses must build rapport; this requires the nurse to be dependable so that the patient can trust that he or she will do what they said they would do (Travelbee 1963). This trust and confidence can be developed along with the sense that the nurse genuinely cares for the patient and cares about what will happen to her or him (Travelbee 1971). In her writings, Travelbee emphasized that when we work to develop trust between the nurse and patient, relationships grow deeper and move from our initial encounter as strangers through the stages of emerging identities (exploring), sympathy (feeling for), empathy (feeling with), and on toward nurse-patient rapport where a true connection is established (Alligood 2018), as seen in Figure 3.1.

This is critically important in spiritual care because there must be a high level of trust in the nurse in order for the patient to open up about what is truly important in their life and situation. While nursing is already seen by Americans as the most trusted profession (Daily Briefing 2020), the vulnerability of being ill and in the hospital places an emotional burden on the patient that can cause them to be reluctant to open up deeply, especially in the mental health setting (Neathery et al. 2020a; Neathery et al. 2020b). So, nurses need to work to promote an atmosphere of openness and safety, where patients can feel that their trust is warranted, and they can share their doubts, questions, and concerns and expect to be treated with dignity and respect (McSherry and Ross 2010). By truly listening and being open and welcoming, nurses can

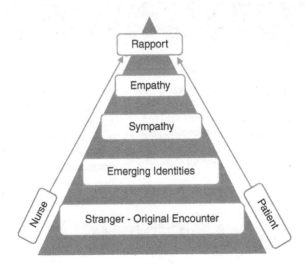

FIGURE 3.1 Travelbee's human-to-human relationship model adapted from resources. *Source*: https://pmhealthnp.com/joyce-travelbee-interpersonal-theory-of-nursing.

identify spiritual concerns, needs, and resources, which is important since everyone has a spiritual nature, but not everyone has a spiritual need.

DETERMINING THE NEED FOR SPIRITUAL CARE

Nurse attitudes are critically important in the facilitation of spiritual care, especially their willingness to be open and vulnerable to their patients (Minton et al. 2018). In a study of nurses from many parts of health services, the authors developed a model (Figure 3.2) that shows how nurses recognize and follow up on spiritual issues. This was a grounded theory study (Artinian et al. 2009) where the main concern of the participants is identified and the resolution of their concern reveals the basic social

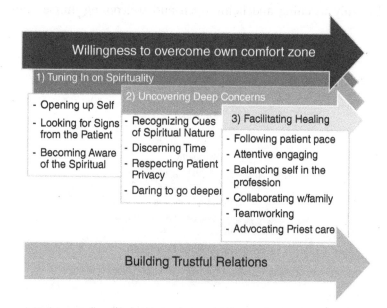

FIGURE 3.2   Discerning the healing path (Giske and Cone 2015/ John Wiley & Sons).

process and emergent theory. In this study, the nurses' main concern was to somehow alleviate the pain, suffering, and other difficulties that their patients were facing. What emerged from the study is that nurses resolved this concern through a three-phase process of *Discerning the healing path* (Giske and Cone 2015) shown in Figure 3.2.

In the first phase, the student or nurse "tunes in" to the patient and tries to discern if there are spiritual concerns, challenges, or perhaps resources that are important for nursing care. When the nurse recognizes expressions of a spiritual nature, she or he goes on to phase two to clarify what it is about. Phase three shows the various aspects that may be relevant in following up with patients in this spiritual domain. Two important conditions must be in place for this process to take place. First, the students/nurses must be willing to go beyond their personal comfort zone if this should be needed, and secondly, they must be able to build and maintain a trusting relationship with the patient, that is, to build and maintain rapport. When these conditions are in place, the process normally begins and moves forward through the three phases (Giske and Cone 2015). The process can develop very quickly or it can take a long time – days, weeks, or even months for those in long-term or out-patient care.

WILLING TO GO OUTSIDE YOUR COMFORT ZONE

In order to understand what is important for the individual patient, students and nurses must be willing to stretch beyond what they are normally comfortable with in patient care (Giske and Cone 2015; Minton et al. 2018). Since talking about spirituality and spiritual issues is perceived by Norwegians as well as many other cultural groups around the world as private and personal, opening up for spiritual, existential, and philosophical concerns can be a challenge for the nurse. Both students and nurses describe this as being willing to go beyond their comfort zone (Cone and Giske 2017; Giske and Cone 2012), in situations like being able to stay fully present with the patient even when feeling tired or overwhelmed, or listening to a patient even if we can feel embarrassed about the topic, feel like we have no answers for the patient, or because we are not used to listening to or talking about spiritual issues. For students, it is often related to developing a professional identity where they can be themselves while at the same time fulfilling their role as a nurse. Many of those we interviewed said that patients want nurses to ask and to truly listen. One student told us that a patient who had pain after a foot operation asked the student to pray for her foot. The student said he could not, but the patient requested it again. The student said that he was thinking about this and was discussing with himself about what it meant to be a nurse. He told us, "So I prayed a little prayer for his foot, because the patient was very anxious" (Giske and Cone 2015, Student Nurse 1).

Being willing to go beyond one's comfort zone is about being open and honest, seeking the person behind the disease or situation, and taking the other person seriously. It means being there for the person and willing to take some risks for the purpose of helping them to get well. It can be about daring to ask questions that may open up a conversation or to listen to the unspoken within a conversation (Minton et al. 2018; Taylor 2007; Ueland 2002). Students and nurses who are willing to go beyond what they are comfortable with know their own vulnerability and that they need personal courage in a professional situation. In order to safeguard both the personal and patient boundaries, it is important to develop a good professional understanding of spirituality and spiritual care.

Reflection 3.1

- Think of one or two professional situations where you were challenged to go beyond your own comfort zone.
- If you did, what concerns made you go outside your comfort zone? How did it turn out?
- When you did not do that, what was your reason? How do you feel about this now?

BUILDING TRUSTING RELATIONSHIPS

The other condition that is needed in order to recognize and follow up existential/spiritual concerns is that the patient experiences having a trusting relationship with the student or the nurse. One of the early things we learn in nursing is about the importance of building rapport and being trusted by our patients. Without such a relationship, healthcare cannot be fully exercised. With highly vulnerable and dependent patients, nurses have great power to contribute to good, constructive relationships or else to promote painful and degrading situations for the patient. Some patients discuss situations and experiences where life feels worthwhile and good, small things have great value, and they are lifted out of the here and now situation to a greater or higher living space. If the relationship is filled with such qualities, the patient knows and confirms it.

This is care that nourishes a person and helps them to continue living, and it stimulates hope and strengthens the patient's life force. This connection with the patient is mutually beneficial to both patient and nurse. Such a positive situation can be identified with big words, but often this is about small and everyday things. A woman we will call Gina was admitted to a hospital and described how the voice, the body language, and the way the nurse spoke clearly and kindly let her know that the nurse was interested in her and wanted to be there. Gina herself spoke of this as spiritual care. In Chapter 1, we briefly discussed caring for the person in a kind and compassionate way (Rykkje et al. 2013) and about the courage required to meet the patient at the point of suffering and to be present together with the patient in that place (Steenfeldt et al. 2018). We interpret this as being what happened here:

Gina: It's about the spiritual or the religious. . .it is difficult to say anything concrete. . .but with humanity. . . I actually experienced this the day before yesterday with a very young nurse . . . I got a message that was very bad and heavy for me. She was just amazing. I can't understand how she could handle it. She was under 25, I think.

> *Researcher:*   What went on?
> *Gina:*   It was the voice, I am very much focused on the voice, I am. It was the voice and the few words she said . . . There weren't many, but she sat next to me here on the bed, and then I had my head on her shoulder and then she held me as long as I wanted. I can't remember what she said, you see. I was the one who spoke the most, but she didn't have any such overwhelming comforting words . . . or . . . it was just the way she was.
>   (Bøe 1999, p. 78)

Nurses say that meeting a patient and a relative with a smile, a touch, or offering some tea or coffee to the next of kin when they are visiting. . .it all matters. Creating an environment in which the patient and relatives feel that the nurse has time and is interested in them builds trusting relationships. In another study, one nurse talked about the fact that "opening up the *inner door* to others" was important because then you are truly opening up to the other (Cone and Giske 2012, Nurse 1). The example above is a concrete one on how a young nurse built such a relationship by daring to be with Gina in a painful life situation even when he had no answers.

In the same way, nighttime situations provide opportunities for deeply personal care, or there can be small things that are experienced as invading patients or decreasing their dignity. The experience of not being truly seen or appreciated can be more about having value than about time. Such a meeting can diminish patient strength and prey on their life force; it can reinforce a sense of emptiness, hopelessness, and of being worthless. Moreover, this negative relationship can take inner confidence away. One patient we will call Rita tells her story this way:

> Yes, I sometimes think – it is . . . [Crying] In a way, it becomes a suffering in itself – an extra offense . . . When they come in here at night, then – is it – yes, there is a mean way, but there are some who say: "What do

you want!" They know very well what I want, but it's the way they say it. I think it's so bad – "WHAT IS IT YOU WANT!"

What does this do to you?

It sounds so brutal – so rough. Those who come in here and do not say "Good night!" Or they do not say "Good morning!" Yes, I will turn away from them. . . I lie awake a long time before I get to sleep afterwards.

(Hovdenes 1998, p. 59, translated by T. Giske)

Even with our best intentions, we fail at times. We may feel that we are crossing boundaries we do not see or could not foresee were there. When a number of students in an early study were interviewed about spirituality and spiritual care, they gave a wide variety of responses. One student in a focus group interview we had told us about an experience from clinical practice:

It was Sunday and I asked one of the patients I was responsible for whether or not they would like to go to the hospital chapel service; it was a most sacred time there. . . It was just a question, but I felt Wilma's response was, "You shouldn't have asked me, I have no interest in it!" Luckily, we could talk about it afterwards when I asked about what happened, so it didn't damage our relationship.

(Giske and Cone 2012, Student 2)

This story led to some reflection in the focus group and others thought that it might be difficult to distinguish between the patients who appreciated being asked about spiritual concerns and those who experience it as offensive. Trusting relationships can break down in different parts of the process, and we must at all times be mindful of how we can build trust and maintain it and not destroy it (Taylor 2007). Nurses and students can develop greater intuition about the time and place for such conversations and learn how to build deeper patient-nurse rapport with increased knowledge, experience, and reflection (Cone and Giske 2020).

Reflection 3.2

- Consider the stories of Gina, Rita, and Wilma. How would you have responded in these situations?
- Think of one or more patients you have been responsible for lately. How did you build a relationship of trust together?
- Did any challenges arise during the relationship? What were these and how did you and the patient handle them?
- Have you experienced that the relationship of trust with a patient was broken? What happened? How did it affect your nursing care for this patient?

TUNING IN TO THE SPIRITUAL DOMAIN

The first phase in the process of discerning the patient's healing path is about being able to recognize spiritual expressions in the patients; this is important for determining if there is a need to be met or a resource that is available or the patient needs help accessing. The students say it is right to do so: "It is important that we are open and think that it can actually happen that for some of our patients' spiritual/existential/religious relationships are important and thus it must be important for us," said one student (Giske and Cone 2012). It is crucial to use patient cues (Steenfeldt et al. 2018) and to open both the ears and the heart so that we can capture what lies there as perhaps an ambiguous hint, an opportunity to provide supportive care (Minton et al. 2018). One nurse said that she lets herself respond to a "gut feeling," which is her intuition; it is enough to make her stop or go deeper (Giske and Cone 2015). One student said:

> It is important to listen to the non-verbal language, because it is really deep for many to talk about such questions. So, you need time and peace and attention to be there for them. People are so different, so you have to be open and talk to them when they want it and don't push them.
>
> (Giske and Cone 2012, Student 3)

Judgment and discernment on signs that may stop a nurse from going deeper can be patients' facial expressions when they lie in bed that show they are unwell or angry, or that they cannot get to sleep or they feel like crying. Nurses who are tuned in to patients notice what patients are asking, as with the "What will happen to me?" questions related to suffering or to death and dying. It is just as much the way in which patients say things that makes the nurse feel that there are some things worth investigating more closely. An experienced nurse said that she had learned to read those little signs in a human face and to use them to help her recognize cues to things that are deeply important to the patient.

Other more visible expressions that can justify the student/ nurse in relation to the attitude of the patient can be the books, pictures, or jewelry we see, or the food and customs they have, as well as what they are talking about or watching on TV. Both students (Giske and Cone 2012) and nurses (Cone and Giske 2013) say that talking about spiritual concerns is taboo in many cultures, and that spirituality truly is very personal and private. Therefore, it is important that they move on very carefully to the next phase, which is about uncovering and understanding more of what they have gotten a sense of from patient cues.

Reflection 3.3

Think of a couple of situations where you became aware of expressions that could be about something spiritual/existential.

- What did you feel like avoiding?
- Were you open for discussion about this? Or did you feel this would cross a boundary?
- Are you usually open for spiritual/existential/religious matters that are important for patients under your care? If not, think about why this may be so.

In the rest of this chapter, we will use storytelling examples to demonstrate how the three phases we refer to in Figure 3.2 can play out in clinical practice. The first story is about Anna Olsen (fictitious name), who was hospitalized for almost two weeks because pneumonia had aggravated her heart failure so that she could no longer cope with home care.

> Anna Olsen is 83 years old and was admitted to the hospital with pneumonia and worsening heart failure 12 days before. She knew herself to be in very poor condition and struggled to breathe when she was admitted. Anna lives "in the countryside" together with her husband and has homecare nursing every other week. At the hospital, she received antibiotics and pulmonary treatment and is now able to take care of herself with help. She manages to sit up in a chair by the bed, all the time connected to O_2. Saliva and other particulates are often troublesome, so suction is frequently needed. She is in a 3-bed room and will soon be ready to go back out into the world. On the morning of the 12th day that Anna was in the hospital, the nurse noticed tears running down Anna's cheeks. At the same time, she smiled. The nurse was confused by the two apparently opposing expressions on Anna's face.

Reflection 3.4

- What do you think about the observations of the nurse?
- What do you suppose is going on with Anna?
- How would you respond if you were the nurse in this situation?

UNVEILING IMPORTANT CONCERNS

Phase two in Figure 3.2 goes on to the processes that students and nurses use to, in a respectful way, uncover and understand more of what is important for patients and their families. This process may require courage to dare to stay in a situation that is unresolved and where you may not have any answers. It requires inner strength to remain in process until we understand more of what is at stake for our patients.

In this clarification process, the nurses listen for two conditions that help them understand how the patient is doing and how they can help. First, they listen to what patients are reporting, how they talk, and what their concern is really about. To judge when a patient is feeling down or is suffering, they try to find out what lies behind the actual words. Topics that nurses recognize as spiritual are expressions of shame, guilt, indulgence, loss and grief, or hope vs hopelessness, or questions about heaven and hell, and questions in relation to faith and rituals. The other relationship nurses seek to understand is the deeply held beliefs that the patient has, especially related to health. Those looking and listening for religious expressions that show what the patient likes mention that patients may include God, Jesus, or prayer in the conversation, and perhaps there are pictures, books, or jewelry that can give hints about what view of life the patient has. Some nurses comment that patients from other countries often experience a more systematic data collection of spiritual needs and resources than patients from Norway (Cone and Giske 2017).

This clarification process, which can go quickly or may take a long time, requires the nurse to consider how to use and allocate the time so that patients who need nursing care the most can receive it, and so that the time is spent in an effective way. In the USA, the admission assessment has a mandated question about faith tradition/religious preferences, but there is no real spiritual assessment at that time, nor are spiritual resources considered. This must be done in the unit by the bedside nurse, so all nurses need to learn how to assess both needs and resources that patients may have in the spiritual domain (Puchalski 2013).

One should also be prepared for when the patient is ready to open up and talk. It is important to respect the patient's boundaries and processes, so being on time, remaining present, and being engaged with them is of great importance because spiritual concerns are deep and personal. A trusting relationship must be in place, and nurses must be willing to go beyond what they are comfortable with to arrive at clarification of what is at stake in the patient's life (Steenfeldt et al. 2018). It usually does not take long; it is mostly about timing and place, as well as the will and courage to go deeper. Many nurses say that it helps them try to get into the patient's situation, that thinking about what they might need if they were a patient helps them to understand and to be courageous (Giske and Cone 2015). Active listening and being quiet together with the patient can be all that is necessary (Minton et al. 2018). For some of us, it may require a great deal of courage, especially in mental health settings (Van Nieuw Amerongen-Meeuse et al. 2020).

The art of asking questions comes into play here. Over time, nurses can gather a series of good basic questions, but learning to ask the right questions at the right time can only develop by trying and failing. This is where the 2Q-SAM is useful because it is a simple and open approach to initiating a conversation about spirituality (Ross and McSherry 2018). Inspiration and guidance about your approach can come from survey interviews developed for student use in practice situations. In Chapter 2, we showed the data collection guides of Ruth Stoll (1979), as well as the FICA (Puchalski 2013) and HOPE (Anandarajah and Hight 2001) interview tools. These can provide structure and help us gain an overview of what we know about and when we need more data. In a study on how comfortable nurses were to do spiritual data collection and to consider spiritual concerns (Cone and Giske 2017), the 172 nurses who participated in the study ranked these questions highest:

1. Who or what supports you when you are sick?
2. What helps you most when you are sick?
3. Do you have spiritual/existential needs or concerns that I can help you with?
4. Do you have anyone you can talk to about religious matters?

Among the participants in the study, 133 of the nurses from all parts of the health services, also gave responses about the questions they used in their own practice. We categorized them into five main groups, and here we list the most commonly used questions in the main group (Cone and Giske 2017):

1. What do you need?
   - What are you thinking about?
   - What is important to you now?
2. Who and what helps you?
   - Is there anyone you would like to talk to?
   - How can we help/support you?

3. Death and the dying process:
   - Are you thinking of death?
   - Are you afraid of dying?
4. Religious clarification:
   - Do you have a belief that helps you or is important to you?
   - Are there religious or spiritual things that you need help with?
5. Religious follow-up:
   - Do you want to talk to a priest/deacon/spiritual leader?
   - What songs do you like?
   - Do you need help reading from the Bible, prayers, or the like?

Reflection 3.5

Think of a couple of situations where you discovered or clarified spiritual/existential/ religious needs and/or resources in your patients.

- Where did this happen and for how long a time did it occur?
- What was it about? What spiritual/existential/religious themes were brought up?
- What questions helped to clarify the situation?
- Were you challenged to go beyond what you are comfortable with? If so, what was this like for you?
- How was your relationship with the patient affected? To what extent did the patient already trust you? Think about what made this trust remain.

Let us go back to the story about Anna Olsen and continue where the nurse became confused by the nonverbal expressions and wondered about the tears that ran down Anna's cheeks and her face that smiled at the nurse. The following dialogue between the nurse and Anna developed:

Nurse: Anna, I see that you smile, but tears run down your cheeks to your chin. . .

Anna answered: I always smile – I have learned it. But inside me, I cry all the time.

(The nurse took her hand, and Anna accepted and she held it firmly.)

Nurse: Anna, can I be allowed to ask you a bit more about this?

Anna: Yes, it is fine

The nurse continued: Do you want to tell a little more about how it is for you right now?

Anna: I have a large lump inside me that lies and weighs heavily in me. I grew up in a Christian family, but my father was so strict and treated us badly. Therefore, I have not had anything to do with Christianity since I was young. I got married and had children, but I have had little contact with them after they were grown. Some years ago, we moved from the city to the countryside where we are now. Because I have gotten so sick, I do not come out and do not have any contact with anyone other than home health nurses who came to us two weeks after my earlier hospitalization.

I haven't told anyone about what it was like in my childhood, so my husband doesn't know anything about this or how I feel now. I have managed to hold on to this turmoil for many years, but now the pain inside me has become so big that I am unable to cope with it anymore! In the ambulance on the way to the hospital, I asked God if He would help me make it to this hospital and that I had to get help with this burden, because it has become completely overwhelming for me!

Nurse:	You say you grew up in a Christian home, but that you have distanced yourself from all that. Do you have anything that helps you now?
Anna:	Yes, I have taken a distance from everything, but I have experienced several times in my life that God has been near and concretely helped me. And I have a little hope that it can happen again. . . .

The nurse recorded that the conversation had taken less than 10 minutes and that she had gotten a pretty good understanding of how Anna feels. It was in the middle of the open morning room, and she had to go do rounds and make the room ready for the breakfast service that would soon start. . .

Reflection 3.6

- What do you think about the way the nurse went forward with Anna to understand what was important to her? Do you feel this revealed Anna's most important concerns?
- Do you see how the nurse listened to the two conditions we presented in the text above:
- What is the patient's report of beliefs?
- What view of life does the patient have?
- Anna came to the hospital with a wish to get help and has been waiting for this for 12 days. Do you have suggestions for how this could have been addressed earlier?
- How can you help ensure that patients receive the help they need, including mental and spiritual care when they receive nursing care?

FACILITATING THE HEALING PROCESS

The transition between clarifying spiritual needs and resources (phase two) and following up a patient (phase three) can be very fluid, because listening and being together with the patient in the clarification process can be of great help. American nursing professor and writer Verna Carson summarizes three ways we can follow up on patients' spiritual issues. They are easy to remember and can make a checklist for us (Carson 2011; Koenig et al. 2012). Many times, we will use these three areas simultaneously.

1. *Being present with.* Being together and fully present with the patient is about attentive presence, about being sensitive, being able to listen actively, relying on quietness and even silence, showing empathy, accepting one's own and the other's vulnerability, and being engaged in the situation. Being alone can be very painful, and dying alone is one of the things that patients really fear when nearing the end of their lives. Presence is one of the most important gifts we can give patients when they are feeling vulnerable and alone or distressed. Touch is also very important at this time. When feeling alone and lonely, people gain strength and hope simply from a touch on the hand or shoulder. So, if nurses can sit down and reach out to touch the patient, even being fully present does not take a long time.

2. *Listening/talking.* Hearing with both ears, in other words, hearing the meaning as well as the words, is one of the most important parts in the process of building trust with our patients. Listening in a non-judgmental manner is important; we must show respect and treat the patient with dignity as we listen. Words can be of great help; we can talk with patients to clarify matters or share thoughts and experiences; however, we must be sure to listen to their answers, paying attention to both verbal and nonverbal language. In the same way as with Anna in the story, there are some patients who find it easier to talk to a nurse or chaplain/priest about spiritual issues than with the family or friends.

If the nurse and the patient have a good relationship, but it is not natural for the nurse to pray, then the nurse may be able to sit with the patient while the patient is praying. As a reminder, listening is more important than talking; shared silence can be very supportive and healing. In addition, it is not necessary to know or have all the answers; you just need to listen and be kind and genuine.

3. *Acting*. The third aspect is about taking action, which often involves making practical arrangements of various kinds. Reading from devotional books, hymn books, or other religious texts can provide encouragement and strength. Some workplaces have created a small resource library in relation to the patient groups they serve, so they have something tangible to use when needed. Patients may experience strength and hope through prayer. In relation to prayer, it is important to examine and identify what the patient wants to ask and to find out what kind of prayer the patient is used to. Some people think that prayer is pre--formulated, such as the *Lord's Prayer* (the *Our Father*), while others are used to a freestyle prayer where you tell God what is in your heart. Others just want to be prayed for quietly or silently. Many nurses feel that it is not right to pray for a patient if they do not share the patient's faith or view of life, but they can simply sit and provide presence while the patient or someone else prays. Calling for spiritual counselors according to the patient's desire and needs may also be an important measure. For some patients, foods are very important. This can be about what food is important to eat or not eat or how it is prepared, and for some, there are serious consequences if their normal practices are not followed. The placement of the bed in the room can be important for Muslims who are bedridden so that they can face Mecca when they pray. In some cultures and religions, there are rules about who can awaken and care for men or women, and especially in relation to ritual washing of the dead; it is important that this is done in the right way and by the right people. Use of symbolic clothing and covering

of body parts can also be important for some. Gaining good general knowledge about different beliefs and life-views can be of great help in our work as nurses since people with different outlook than one's own are found everywhere in the world (Taylor 2012; Horsfjord 2017); it is especially important to have knowledge of different rites at end-of-life (Plesner and Døvig 2009). We want to emphasize that cooperation with the patient and family is very important so that the best possible facilitation in relation to what is desirable and optimal for the individual patient can be accomplished.

When we look at the third phase of the model in Figure 3.2, we see that the first point is about following the patient's pace (Giske and Cone 2015). Whatever we do to help, it is crucial that it happens at the patient's wishes and that we gently let the patient lead us. Most patient situations are not acute, so following the patient's process at their own pace is the best way to go. However, even when a situation is acute or the patient is in crisis, the nurse must be careful to go at the patient's pace and not force dialogue and/or decisions. The patient must be respected and we must remain aware that the trust between the nurse and the patient is vitally important.

In our study of nurses, we identified a construct that we call "attentively engaged" (Giske and Cone 2015), which Minton et al. (2018) also found in their study. This construct means that nurses pay attention so that they can tailor appropriate measures based on their professional judgment about what can be good and can help their patients. It may be quiet time together with the patient, while they listen or ponder, or it may mean sitting and listening with full engagement to what the patient is trying to express. It may also involve asking questions, singing with or for the patient, praying with or for the patient, or simply paying attention to what and when the patient asks something of us. It can also be to facilitate time for the patient and the family so that their last time together becomes as worthwhile and precious as possible. Sometimes this is done in person, but it can also be done virtually, as was often the case during the recent pandemic, when in-person presence of the family is not possible.

Nurses know that in situations where patients are severely ill or dying, the family and relatives are particularly vulnerable. The family may need information and teaching as well as concrete advice and help to learn how to act and behave when life comes to an end. Being invited in and given time and space so that the family and relatives can spend time to say goodbye is important. Many nurses commented that relatives who did not have any religious background seemed to be more helpless in meeting with dying patients and that it looked like the lack of rituals made it difficult to find ways of connecting and making sense of the situation (Giske and Cone 2015).

In the work of following up patients' spiritual/existential/religious needs and resources, you must find out how to balance what/who you are as a person with what is needed as a professional nurse in the situation. The nurse, with her or his knowledge, strength, and vulnerability, embraces how a nurse works and meets patients and relatives. Facilitating spiritual care is especially challenging when the patient and the nurse have different beliefs. Here we have to find out what it means to help the patient in a respectful manner while at the same time being sincere and true to self as well as to the patient.

Cooperation in the team where you work is important for the exercise of spiritual care. By using the diversity of resources in the team and by using each individual's special expertise, the nurse can provide the best patient follow-up. If one is not comfortable meeting patients with different beliefs, then a team that knows each other will be open to referrals, within and beyond the team, and together they can find out how to be of best help. Our earlier discussion on general and special competencies is important to remember. While we do not want to simply pass a patient who has different beliefs off to another team member, there may be times when this is truly the best option for both patient and nurse. For example, if the patient wants a nurse to pray and the nurse does not feel comfortable doing so, then the nurse can suggest sitting and being present with the patient during the prayer or calling a nurse who is comfortable praying. The patient can decide which they prefer. This can actually strengthen the trust relationship if handled carefully and respectfully.

Documentation of spiritual concerns is also important for continuity in the follow-up of patients. In follow-up reports from nurses, Giske et al. (2018) report that hostile relationships are often neither discussed in the verbal report nor documented in the nursing notes on the patient charts. This is something that challenges both the individual nurse and the healthcare team to ensure that spiritual care is the same standard as the rest of the nursing care. Clear, unambiguous nurses' notes are important to promote consistency as well as continuity of care.

Being able to refer the patient to others can be good nursing care. Some patients want to talk to people other than those who are at the hospital, and if the patient or family needs help contacting this person, the nurse must facilitate that. For patients with a different life-view than the Christian, the patient or family will usually know who to contact. If there is uncertainty about this, nurses can contact the hospital chaplaincy for their help in identifying beliefs and life-views, and they will help to get in touch with the appropriate spiritual leaders.

When nurses have discovered that patients are struggling with spiritual issues, they often recommend that the patient can have a conversation with a priest/hospital chaplain. The nurses in our study had great confidence that a chaplain will show respect for and can help patients with different beliefs. Many say the chaplain/priest is good at listening and has time for patients who need it. Because patients may think that they are seriously ill or dying if there is talk of a priest, the nurse tries to normalize a conversation with the hospital chaplain and portray it as routine to meet with this branch of the healthcare team (Giske and Cone 2015; Cone and Giske 2017). Now, let us return to the story about Anna and look at the follow-up on the 12th day of her hospitalization:

> The nurse realized that during that morning conversation she had gained insight into a part of what was important for Anna and the beliefs she has. Anna would soon be going back out into the world, so time was short to get help for the inner pain Anna is praying about. Anna has not told her family about how it has been for her through

the years, so the nurse decided not to involve the family at this time.

The nurse said:	Anna, I think it is brave of you to tell me about what is so difficult for you. As you know, you have benefited from the treatment here and you will soon be discharged to go home to your husband. The time is short, so I would suggest that you talk with a competent person here at the hospital about your inner pain. My experience is that our hospital chaplain is a good and wise conversation partner, and he has more time than nurses here on the ward. If you think it is okay, I will contact him this morning so he can come to you today.
Anna:	Yes, it's probably okay, you can do it.
The nurse:	That's good. I will contact him with a time so he can start come see you today.

Reflection 3.7

- What do you think about the way the nurse did follow-up with Anna?
- Do you have other suggestions for what to do?
- How would you report this conversation in the oral report and what would you document in the written nurses' notes? Justify your answer.

DOCUMENTING SPIRITUAL CONCERNS

As we pointed out in Chapter 1, spiritual care is part of the nurse's responsibility, and it is one of the areas in the electronic healthcare documentation system that can be identified as "specialist health services." It is noted as part of NANDA (2016) diagnoses, and some documentation systems actually have a code for cultural and lifestyle issues, spiritual life concerns, and spiritual well-being or distress. The fact that we use this point for assessment, planning, intervention/implementation, and evaluation and follow-up of spiritual care for patients when relevant helps to emphasize that spiritual care is not a private but a professional relationship. In nursing, we often use scripted documentation to visualize what is important for the patient and what has been done, but some things need to be described in comment areas. Accurate and complete nursing documentation ensures that what is to be followed up is made clear to everyone who works with the patient 24/7. If spiritual/existential concerns that are of importance to the patient are not documented, they will simply disappear when the person who has been with the patient goes off duty. Written documentation of spiritual care is particularly important for the working environment in which a silent or non-verbal report has been introduced.

One of the reasons why nursing notes rarely report on spiritual concerns can be that the nurse feels that this is very personal to the patient and that we can thus be uncertain about how we should write up what has gone on with the patient. These are important factors to think about so that we take care of the patient's integrity in the documentation. In some places today, there are hospitals where patients can log in and read their own healthcare journal. This reminds us that we must always document with care so that the patient feels that what we write is correct and that it communicates that nursing has provided the best possible care for the patient. If we are uncertain, in most cases we can ask the patient to affirm what we write in the nursing documentation to ensure that it is accurate and that the patient receives good follow-up.

So, how could we formulate a written report on Anna Olsen to make sure that she would receive good follow-up in the spiritual area that had been waiting for 12 days? Here is our suggestion showing that Anna struggled with something, without explaining what it was. The report also says that the hospital chaplain had established contact. If for some reason the hospital chaplain does not follow up, then the nurse who is responsible for Anna has the opportunity to catch this missing step and do something about it. This brief report also states that others who read it will understand that there is more in Anna's life than heart failure and pneumonia.

> In the morning assessment, it emerged that Anna was struggling with thoughts that were worse after getting pneumonia. When it was clear that she would soon be ready for discharge, the hospital chaplain was contacted for an appointment with Anna. He had a first conversation with her today and will follow up as long as she is at the hospital. Nursing needs to facilitate that the chaplain and Anna can converse in a sheltered and quiet place where they will not be overheard.

Reflection 3.8

- What do you think is important to document about spiritual care? Should it be done in the same way as physical and psychosocial care?
- Have you documented anything about spiritual concerns of your patients?
- If yes, what was it about?
- If you did not, what was your reasoning?
- How would you formulate the written documentation about Anna Olsen?

DIFFERENT CONDITIONS THAT AFFECT SPIRITUALITY

In this chapter, we have seen how one can assess, recognize, and follow up on spiritual health, existential needs, and resources in patients. We will end by looking at different conditions that can affect this process. We will briefly address four conditions: (1) the nurse, (2) the patient, (3) the patient's family, and (4) the working environment (Giske and Cone 2015).

First of all, how comfortable nurses are with their own spirituality affects, to a certain extent, whether and how they see spiritual care as part of overall nursing care (Cone and Giske 2017;

Giske and Cone 2015; Ross et al. 2016). Nurses who are at peace within themselves, regardless of their belief system, are the most comfortable with spiritual care giving (Cone 1997). By pursuing personal and professional growth and development, nurses can deepen and broaden our ability to facilitate patient-centered spiritual care. Nurses and patients do not always see eye to eye on spiritual issues or on health beliefs, so building trustful relationships with patients will make a difference in how easily we can make connections at a deep level (Giske and Cone 2020). Interactions between patients and students/nurses are also influenced by how long-term a relationship they may have. In the health services, there are many short meetings, such as in the ambulance, emergency room, admitting area, or in and out of the operating theaters. We recommend that you develop a conscious relationship with time so that you are more aware and intentional in its use. The fact that time is short does not mean that spiritual care cannot find a place; in fact, it is the nurse's genuinely caring attitude that carries the most weight in these brief encounters.

Thinking about the patient, it is important to consider the patient's age, if they are growing older, whether or not there are children, and to what extent they have the language to talk about spiritual concerns. It may also be a deciding factor in how the care and follow-up is done if the patient is acutely or chronically ill. There is a great deal of unanimity among healthcare providers that patients who are in the palliative and/or terminal phase are more open and aware of spiritual concerns than other patient groups (Nolan et al. 2011). To what extent patients perceive their situation as a crisis and how willing they are to open up to healthcare personnel will influence how easily these deep concerns come to the fore. Since trust is important, it is often easier to find time and space both for assessment and follow-up when the relationship lasts over time as it often does in nursing homes and in-home care. Things and symbols such as books, pictures, jewelry, and other visual cues can provide information about the patient's life, interests, and values, but we want to emphasize that it is important to confirm what this means to the patient. One nurse said in an interview: "The house looked like a church, but that meant nothing to the patient" (Giske and Cone 2015, Nurse 2), noting that her patient had simply held on to the things that were precious to his mother. What patients watch on TV, what food they eat, whether they attend special meetings or church can help the nurse understand more of who the individual patient is and what is important to them. Many nurses say that certain ethnic patients are less open and more reserved in relation to spiritual care than patients from other cultures or ethnic groups. However, they see the same spiritual concerns in all patients; it is only that the cultural packaging is different (Giske and Cone 2015; Cone and Giske 2017), so focusing on the individual patient is vital.

Thirdly, relationships around patients are very important; the patient's family has great meaning, and nurses often work with relatives and extended family members. Family values and beliefs as well as knowledge of and insight into the patient's situation affect this collaboration. Parents are often not ready to accept that their child will die, and they may not allow the nurse to talk to the child about death; family wishes can be a barrier or a facilitator. When patients are critically ill or dying, nurses know that relatives are particularly vulnerable to what is being said, and they can positively or negatively affect the mourning process. If there is a sudden death or a suicide, the nurse's main focus is the family and how to support them in the best possible way so they can move along their journey through grief and loss (Neathery et al. 2020b).

The fourth condition is the workplace environment. Number of employees, time allowed for each patient, having a heavy patient load or being in a hurry in the department or as a work team, and the pace or rhythm of different shifts all set limits on interactions and relationships with patients (Koenig 2013). These factors affect how nurses can lead, seek knowledge, plan care, and discuss and report on spiritual issues, conversations, and relationships with colleagues. The workplace environment promotes spiritual care as an integrated and natural part of the follow-up of patients when it is a topic of internal teaching, is discussed in reports, and is the topic of interdisciplinary meetings where the chaplain or priest/deacon/spiritual leader (philosophy of life) is part of the team

(Van Nieuw Amerongen-Meeuse et al. 2020). The opposite of such openness in the team is an unwelcoming environment where it is not seen as relevant or is even prohibited to discuss spiritual or religious themes. Therefore, ongoing professional development needs to include increasing knowledge on various religions and life-views, especially as they relate to health.

Reflection 3.9

Choose a situation you have recently experienced in which spiritual concerns emerged. Think about how the four conditions we have discussed affect what happened between you and the patient and possibly the relatives.

- What conditions promoted that spiritual concerns came up and were followed up?
- What conditions of the patient and the family had particular significance?
- How did the working environment affect what happened? To what extent did you have support from the leader and/ or colleague?

FROM CONNECTION TO REFLECTION

This chapter on connecting with patients has covered the importance of building rapport between the nurse and patient, recognizing if there is a need for spiritual care, discerning the healing path through moving outside your comfort zone and building trust into your relationships and being "tuned in" to the spiritual domain. We have discussed ways to ask questions and shown how the use of genuine compassionate care can enable you to reach and touch patients deeply and support them through difficult times toward healing and wholeness. We also spent a little time on the importance of documenting spiritual care in a respectful yet clear way so that others can follow up on the care we provide. While there are a number of conditions that can positively or negatively affect the work of nurses, we hope our suggestions can help you to promote a healthy and healing environment, though that will be discussed further in our concluding chapter. We ended with some tips for nurses who supervise students in clinical practice, which is of great importance since students often say they lack role models for spiritual care. Chapter 4 is where we discuss the process of reflecting on what we have done. It is very important to think about our actions, both when we do well and when we could have done better. This will move us on in our personal and professional growth as nurses who facilitate spiritual care.

REFERENCES

Alligood, M.R. (ed.) (2018). *Nursing Theorists and their Work*, 9ee. Mosby Elsevier.

Anandarajah, G. and Hight, E. (2001). Spirituality and medical practice: using the HOPE questions as a practical tool for spiritual assessment. *American Family Physician* 63 (1): 81–89.

Artinian, B., Giske, T., Cone, P.H., and (Eds.). (2009). *Glaserian Grounded Theory in Nursing Research: Trusting Emergence*. Springer.

Bøe, K.G. (1999). *Åndelig omsorg – sanselig nærvær* (Hovedoppgåve) [Spiritual care – sensory presence] (Master Thesis). Det teologiske fakultet, Universitetet i Oslo.

Carson, V.B. (2011). What is the essence of spiritual care? *Journal of Christian Nursing* 28 (3): 173.

Cone, P. (1997). Connecting: the experience of giving spiritual care. In: *The Intersystem Model: Integrating Theory and Practice* (ed. B.M. Artinian and M. Conger). Sage Publications.

Cone, P.H. and Giske, T. (2013). Teaching spiritual care: a grounded theory study among undergraduate nursing educators. *Journal of Clinical Nursing* 22 (13–14): 1951–1960. https://doi. org/10.1111/j.1365-2702.2012.04203.x.

Cone, P.H. and Giske, T. (2017). Nurses' comfort level with spiritual assessment: a mixed method study among nurses working in diverse healthcare settings. *Journal of Clinical Nursing* 26 (19–20): 3125-3136. https://doi.org/10.1111/jocn.13660.

Daily Briefing (2020). For the 18th year in a row, nurses are the most-trusted profession, according to Gallup. https://www.advisory.com/daily-briefing/2020/01/10/nurse-trusted (accessed 22 March 2022).

Giske, T. (2012). How undergraduate nursing students learn spiritual care in clinical studies – a review of literature. *Journal of Nursing Management* 20: 1049–1057.

Giske, T. and Cone, P.H. (2012). Opening up for learning: a grounded theory study of nursing student education on spiritual care. *Journal of Clinical Nursing* 21 (13–14): 2006–2015.

Giske, T. and Cone, P.H. (2015). Discerning the healing path: how nurses assist patients spiritually in diverse healthcare settings. *Journal of Clinical Nursing* 24: 10–20. 10.111/jocn.12907.

Giske, T., & Cone, P.H. (2020). Comparing nurses' and patients' comfort level with spiritual assessment. *Religions 2020* 11 (12): 671. [Special Issue "Spirituality in Healthcare—Multidisciplinary Approach"] https://doi.org/10.3390/rel11120671.

Giske, T., Melås, S.N., and Einarsen, K.A. (2018). The art of oral handover: a participant observational study by undergraduate students in a hospital setting. *Journal of Clinical Nursing* 27 (5–6): e767–e775. https://doi.org/10.1111/jocn.14177.

Horsfjord, V. (2017). *Religion I Praksis [Religion in Practice]*. Universitetsforlaget.

Hovdenes, G.H. (1998). *Et meningsfylt liv i sykehjemmet: "vennlighet først og sist": en fenomenologisk studie av sykehjemsbeboeres opplevelse av mening i livet.* (Hovedfagsoppgåve) [A meaningful life in the nursing home: "Kindness first and foremost": A phenomenological study of nursing home residents' experience of meaning in life (Master's thesis)]. Universitetet i Bergen.

Koenig, H.G. (2013). *Spirituality in Patient Care: Why, How, When, and What*, 3ee. Templeton Foundation Press https://doi.org/10.1177/0898010115580236.

Koenig, H.G., King, D., and Carson, V.B. (2012). *Handbook in Religion and Health*. Oxford University Press.

May, R. (1953). Religion—Source of strength or weakness? *Pastoral Psychology* 4: 68–74. https://doi.org/10.1007/BF01786367.

McEwen, M. and Wills, E.M. (2017). *Theoretical Frameworks for Nursing*, 5ee. Lippincott Williams & Wilkens.

McSherry, W. and Ross, L. (2010). *Spiritual Assessment in Healthcare Practice*. M & K Publishing.

Minton, M.E., Isaacson, M.J., Varilek, B.M. et al. (2018). A willingness to go there: nurses and spiritual care. *Journal of Clinical Nursing* 27 (1–2): https://doi.org/10.1111/jocn.13867.

Neathery, M., He, Z., Taylor, E.J., and Deal, B. (2020a). Spiritual perspectives, spiritual care, and knowledge of recovery among psychiatric mental health nurses. *Journal of the American Psychiatric Association* 26 (4): 364–372. https://doi.org/10.1177/1078390319846548.

Neathery, M., Taylor, E.J., and He, Z. (2020b). Perceived barriers to providing spiritual care among psychiatric mental health nurses. *Archives of Psychiatric Nursing* 34 (6): 572–579. https://doi.org/10.1016/j.apnu.2020.10.004.

Nolan, S., Saltmarsh, P., & Leget, C. (2011). Spiritual care: Working towards an EAPC task force. *European Journal of Palliative Care* 18: 86–89.

North American Nursing Diagnosis Association [NANDA]. (2016). Nursingdiagnoses.http://www.nandanursingdiagnosislist.org (accessed 22 March 2022).

Plesner, I.T. and Døvig, C.A. (Eds.). (2009). *Livsfaseriter – Religions- og livssynspolitiske utfordringer i Norge* [Life phases – Religious and philosophical policy challenges in Norway]. Samarbeidsrådet for tros- og livssyn [The Council for Faith and Beliefs], Oslo.

Puchalski, C.M. (2013). Integrating spirituality into patient care: an essential element of person-centered care. *Polskie Archiwum Medycyny Wewnetrznej* 123 (9): 491–497.

Ross, L. and McSherry, W. (2018). Two questions that ensure person-centred spiritual care. *Nursing Standard.* https://rcni.com/nursing-standard/features/two-questions-ensure-person-centred-spiritual-care-137261 (accessed 22 March 2022).

Ross, L., Giske, T., Van Leeuwen, R. et al. (2016). Factors contributing to student nurses'/midwives' perceived competence in spiritual care: findings from a European pilot study. *Nurse Education Today* 36: 445–451. https://doi.org/10.1016/j.nedt.2015.10.005.

Rykkje, L.R., Eriksson, K., and Råholm, M.B. (2013). Spirituality and caringinoldageandthesignificanceofreligion:ahermeneuticalstudy from Norway. *Scandinavian Journal of Caring Science* 27: 275–284. https://doi.org/10.1111/j.1471-6712.2012.01028.x.

Steenfeldt, V.Ø., Sommer, C., and Wiggers, M.V. (2018). Trialog. *Fag og Forskning* 3: 14–37.

Stoll, R.I. (1979). Guidelines for spiritual assessment. *American Journal of Nursing* 79 (9): 1572–1577.

Taylor, E.J. (2007). *What Do I Say? Talking with Patients about Spirituality*. Templeton Foundation Press.

Taylor, E.J. (ed.) (2012). *Religion: A Clinical Guide for Nurses*. Springer Publishing.

Travelbee, J. (1963). What do we mean by rapport? *American Journal of Nursing* 63 (2): 70–72.

Travelbee, J. (1971). *Interpersonal Aspects of Nursing*, 2ee. F. A. Davis Company.

Ueland, V. (2002). Sykepleieren og den åndelige/eksistensielle samtalen. Hvordan kan vi konkret samtale med pasienten? [the nurse and the spiritual/existential conversation. How can we concretely talk to the patient?]. *Kreftsykepleie* 3: 11–19.

Van Nieuw Amerongen-Meeuse, J.C., Schaap-Jonker, H., Westerbroek, G. et al. (2020). Conversations and beyond: religious/spiritual care needs among clinical mental health patients in the Netherlands. *The Journal of Nervous and Mental Disease* 208 (7): 524–532. https://doi.org/10.1097/NMD.0000000000001150.

CHAPTER 4

Reflecting and Growing Personally and Professionally

The final phase of our learning spiral is reflection. Intentional reflection will move knowledge gained to the deeper pathways in our brain as experience solidifies what we learn (Balgopal and Montplaisir 2011). There are various ways to practice reflection, and by using a variety of strategies, we can identify what works best for us and what helps us learn to apply what we know to various situations that nurses face while caring for patients. The European EPICC Network of spiritual care scholars (see website: www.epicc-network.org) has explored spirituality and health through a broad review of healthcare literature as well as through ongoing research. Over the years, scholars who have learned about spiritual care developed a *Standard of Spiritual Care Competencies* (found on the EPICC website), which we discuss later in this chapter, that can assist nursing students and nurses/midwives to grow in the spirituality and health domain.

The Nurse's Handbook of Spiritual Care, First Edition. Pamela Cone and Tove Giske.
© 2022 John Wiley & Sons Ltd. Published 2022 by John Wiley & Sons Ltd.

Moreover, students as well as practicing nurses can do spiritual self-assessment using the newly developed and recently validated tool (also found on EPICC website) created by the *SEP* (Spiritual care Education and Practice) scholars (Giske et al. 2022). Reflexivity is both an art and a science, and it takes practice to develop competencies through individual and group reflection.

DIMENSIONS AND LEVELS OF REFLECTION

Reflecting means to think about and try to understand the reason for something. It can be done in various ways and on several levels. The American philosopher Donald Alan Schön developed the theory of how critical thinkers teach certain subjects through reflexivity (Schön 1983/2001), and the Swedish philosopher Bengt Molander (2015) explains how we develop knowledge through practical action. Both write about the significance of reflection at different times in relation to a situation. We can reflect on a situation *before* we go into it and imagine what can happen. In this way, we can prepare ourselves with different options for action, and we identify our pre-understanding of the situation. When we are *in* the situation, we can reflect on what is happening while it is happening, something that helps us to actively stay in and be fully present in the situation, to consider what is right or advisable to do, and to act deliberately and intentionally. The last way is to reflect on a situation *after* the event is over. While all of these aspects of reflection are useful and important (Cone and Giske 2018), it is this last form of reflection that we discuss in this chapter (Figure 4.1).

Reflection and reflective writing are useful in every profession; it can be considered a management or leadership skill that will enhance both education and practice (Sen 2010). In education, we use reflection notes or reflection logs to teach students a systematic way of reflecting on their actions and interactions with patients (Cone and Giske 2017). The practice of systematic reflection can help students to become aware of and develop confidence in the professional intuition that they develop through clinical practice (Giske 2012). Moreover, repetition of the reflective process

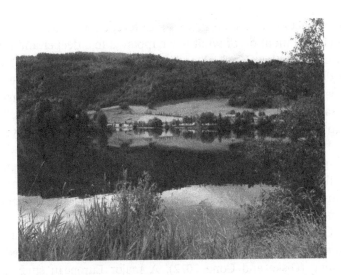

FIGURE 4.1   Reflection: comparison, analysis, and critique.
Source: Photograph of Voss Lake, Norway by Cone.

integrates it into the nurse's natural daily practice. In healthcare services, some established reflection groups meet at an agreed time and place, often with a leader to guide them (Sen 2010), where the staff share experiences and jointly ask and investigate (reflect on) what happened and what one can learn from it. Such systematic reflection in groups is a good way to both work through challenging situations, to learn about difficult subjects, and to develop practical knowledge (Cone and Giske 2018).

What happens when we reflect can be understood in two ways (Hovland and Andresen 2007). The first is that we think through situations and experiences to create meaning about what has happened. Through reflection, we can thus get a deeper understanding of an event (Balgopal and Montplaisir 2011). The other way to understand reflective practices is that reflection after an event gives a certain distance to what has happened. This distance helps us to see ourselves in the situation and thus to get a clearer understanding of how we thought and acted in the situation. It is important to have distance to gain perspective on and overview of what has happened (Molander 2015).

Reflection can take place at different levels from a mere superficial mention of what has happened to a deeper and more critical reflection (Hovland and Andresen 2007; Moon 2007). It is the deeper reflection we want to invite in this chapter, the one that leads to the development of personal competence and change in or transformation of practice (Hovland and Andresen 2007). This deep and critical reflection opens us up to look with new eyes at what has happened so that we see new opportunities we had not thought of earlier. Deep reflection stimulates us to become more familiar with ourselves, the knowledge base we have, the values, meanings, and experiences we have within us, and what we have to build on related to a specific situation.

One study of students showed that thinking through what had happened and sharing experiences with others contributed to learning (Giske and Cone 2012). A major European study also showed that discussions with fellow students were important for the development of spiritual care competence (Ross et al. 2018). Sharing experiences and listening to others' stories even from teachers, fellow students, or directors in practice led the students to be more conscious of their own experience and to get new ideas for how they could act. Such conversations with others also enhance understanding of one's own practice. The students in our study said that discussions with others in a safe environment could increase their degree of comfort for spiritual care (Giske and Cone 2012). To the extent that an environment is known to be safe, group reflection opens us up to share experiences, to put words on feelings, prejudices, and lack of understandings, and to share difficult situations and things that did not go so well (Cone and Giske 2018). Reflexive practice requires that we address both our successful encounters and those that were difficult, challenging, and/or had negative outcomes.

REFLECTING ON WHAT WENT WELL

Thinking about what we did that was useful or helpful to the patient is important because it solidifies the positive attitudes and actions that we do, moving them from intuition to experience, and from there, to part of our personal and professional identity. For example, if we respond in a certain way because it felt like the right thing to do, and it turns out to really help the patient, then the next time we are in a spiritual encounter, we will trust our intuition a little more. By reflecting deeply on the situation and our thoughts, feelings, and actions about it, nurses may be able to recognize the cues that influenced our inner self and to make a note of them so that we can respond in an appropriate way the next time we face a similar situation. Personal and professional growth happens when we reflect on what we did and identify the attitudes and actions that contributed to a positive outcome (Cone and Giske 2013a).

The authors have always believed in whole person care and have looked for ways to help patients who seem to have deep inner struggles. When working as a nurse working in a cancer research hospital many years ago, the first author met a young woman 19 years old (call her Ruth) with non-Hodgkin's lymphoma who was dying because there were no effective cancer treatments at that time. Ruth and her husband (we will call him James) were high school sweethearts who had married as soon as they received the news of her terminal illness. . .

Ruth and James were counting their days together and trying to make precious memories for the young 19-year-old husband who would soon be left alone. I noted on Ruth's chart that they were Christians from the Assembly of God church, which was the same as my own tradition, and they had a belief in divine healing. After completing my assessment of Ruth and noticing the way the two young people clung to each other's hands, I asked them if there was anything I could do to help them with their journey through this illness. James asked if I would pray with them, and Ruth nodded with tears in her eyes.

So, I put my hand over their clasped hands and prayed, "Dear Lord, you see your children Ruth and James, and we know you love them deeply. After all, you died for them! I ask that you hear their hearts' cry and put your healing hand on Ruth. We know from your Word and from our own experience that you do heal people, though not always in the way that we ask. We know that you sometimes use the medical staff and modern medicine to heal, and that you sometimes simply pour your healing power on a person and miraculously bring healing. And we also know that you sometimes choose not to heal but to bring us through the valley of the shadow of death to your home in heaven. But your Word says that sometimes we do not have because we do not ask, so we are asking. We ask for complete healing for Ruth so that she and James can have a happy life together! We believe that you will do what is best and right for James and Ruth, and we trust you completely. So, we will accept from your hand whatever answer you give. We receive it with peace because we know you always act for our good. Thank you Father God, in Jesus' name, Amen."

The faces of James and Ruth were shining with joy as they thanked me. But the nurse supervisor was very angry with me for this prayer because she said it gave the patient "false hope." She went to the hospital leaders, and the administration called me in about this complaint. I told them exactly what happened and what I had said in my prayer. Fortunately, Ruth's physician spoke up for me and said that the patient believed in prayer, had asked me to pray, and that I had not actually promised anything or given false hope, so it was okay to pray if the patient asked for that.

Not long afterwards, Ruth went into spontaneous remission and went home. A year later, she came back with a severe case of the illness, and I cared for her again. Ruth was at peace to be dying, and she thanked me for praying for her because she and James had a very special year together!

Reflection 4.1

- Think about this story and the various outcomes for both Ruth and James.
- What went well in this scenario? What do you think prepared the nurse to act in this way?
- What was the patient outcome (not simply considering the remission) and the family outcome?
- What would you have done in this situation?
- What went wrong or could have gone wrong?

Situations where there are differing beliefs can be very challenging (Neathery et al. 2020b). Many times, patients who were Muslim believers asked for prayer saying they could tell that the nurse/author believed in God, and simply praying to God and asking for His mercy and presence rather than praying according to my own beliefs was completely appropriate and appreciated. In that case, it should not include prayers that were like the situation with Ruth and James where I knew we were on the same page in our beliefs. In one situation, this nurse cared for a patient we will call Hadassah whose chart noted that she was of the Muslim faith. When seeing her deep sadness over her terminal diagnosis, the nurse asked Hadassah if there was anything she could do. The nurse told Hadassah that she was a Christian but that both believe in the Great Creator God and she would be happy to pray as long as Hadassah understood that they were not of the same faith tradition. She said, "We serve the same God in different ways. . ." So, the nurse prayed to Father God for her peace and comfort and for her to feel His presence with her as well as for Him to sustain her on this journey through suffering. She also prayed for comfort for Hadassah's family. They prayed with bowed heads, holding hands, and both said "Amen" at the end. Hadassah tearfully expressed deep gratitude for my prayer.

The nurse's attitude must be open and accepting, and the actions must follow the patient's own beliefs, or at least, not go contrary to their beliefs. At the very least, the nurse can provide presence so that the patient is not alone when they pray or recite something from their own sacred writings. Below is a story told in a research study among Norwegian teachers that exemplifies one aspect of this type of situation. This nurse shared what can happen when there were different beliefs between patient (fictitious name used) and staff:

> I have a great aunt we will call Aunt Beth living in a nursing home that was quite far from me, and I would try to go and visit her every month. Her vision had been failing, and she had limited mobility. One time when I visited Aunt Beth, she was very sad, and when I asked what that was about, she said it was hard to be left alone and not even have God's Word to comfort her (since she could no longer read it herself). I asked Aunt Beth if the nurses did not read to her, and Aunt Beth said "Oh yes, they read the newspaper every morning! But I would love to have a daily Psalm! Would you read one to me today?" So, I read a Psalm to my dear aunt and we sang together and had a nice time, and she was happy.
>
> When I left Aunt Beth, I went to the nurses and asked why they did not read a Psalm from the Bible for my aunt each morning. They replied, "Oh but we do not believe in the Bible!" I said "And you believe in the newspaper?" They were very surprised when I put it that way. I told them that they need to do what the patient asks whenever possible, and they agreed that it was possible to read something they did not believe if the patient wanted them to read something. I hope they are reading a Psalm every day to Aunt Beth!

Reflection 4.2

- Think about this situation and how the nurses treated "Aunt Beth."

- Was Aunt Beth treated with respect? What would you have done?
- What can we do that will respond to different belief systems than our own?
- How can you balance personal and professional roles in a way that respects both the patient and the nurse?

REFLECTING ON WHAT DID NOT GO WELL

It is particularly important to reflect on times where there were difficulties with the situation, it was a demanding or frightening situation, or where we have experienced failure or fear. These types of experiences can make us avoid similar situations later because it was unpleasant for us. For example, there was a patient who appeared anxious and upset, and since her chart noted that she, like the nurse, was "Christian," the nurse asked her if there was something she could do, such as pray with her, or if there was someone the nurse could call for her. She replied, rather angrily, "No, do not bother! God does not listen to me anyhow!" So she said, "I'm so sorry you feel that way. Please let me know if there is anything else you need me to do for you." Having been a nurse for 25 years at that point, that nurse did not let the patient's anger upset her. The nurse thought about what had happened and decided that she simply needed to be kind and caring and to pray for her within herself (exercising her own belief system), and then just let it go. That nurse has stated that she did not let that experience keep her from addressing spiritual issues with other patients after that and that she always tries to be informed and to pay attention to her intuition when addressing deeply personal, important concerns in the spiritual domain.

Through reflection, we have the opportunity to transform demanding and painful experiences into lessons to use in new and similar situations. Here is a sad example that shows how the lack of reflection and learning after a frightening experience prevented the nurse (we will call her Nurse Elsa) from developing better ways to follow up the patients' spiritual issue.

During a collaborative internal staff education session with the hospital chaplain/priest where the themes were meditating, hope, and life-will, an older nurse called Elsa told us she did not talk to patients about private or spiritual issues and she never mentioned hospital priests. The reason for this was that some years ago, Elsa was responsible for a patient feeling upset and uneasy. Elsa had asked the patient if he wanted to talk to the priest, and the patient had so much anxiety over that question that he had almost died! The patient saw this question about the priest as a sign that he was dying, but he was not. Nurse Elsa experienced this as very frightening and she said that after that event, none of the nurses in their unit ever talked to their patients about things related to beliefs or about offering them priests to talk with about their concerns.

Reflection 4.3

- What do you think about the situation the nurse described?
- How could Nurse Elsa have learned from this situation and adjusted her practice?
- What would you do differently, as a nurse or as a nurse leader?

Developing Self-Understanding Through Reflection

Initially, we explained that reflection can be understood in two ways, first about how to create meaning in a patient situation, and secondly about reflection after a situation and how it enhances self-understanding for how to act in a future situation (Hovland and Andresen 2007). As we discussed earlier, the most important single factor for whether and how nurses are "tuned in" to spiritual care is the self-understanding and awareness of the nurse. We present here a way of reflecting on what addresses thoughts, feelings, and choices considered during reflection on how one understands self in a particular situation.

We learned this way of working from pastors in pastoral counseling. These counselors write down situations they will reflect on in a format that shows what has been said and done written in the left column and the inner reflection and dialogue that took place along the way written in the right column. This exercise helps us to become aware of the feelings we have and the choices we make along the way in a situation. Anyone who has learned to work systematically with such reflection can practice changing perspectives between being in the situation and thinking about what is happening in the situation. By being able to move between these two levels while we are in the situation, we can make more thoughtful choices than when we are just in the here and now of the situation and must take time for the reflection afterwards.

We remind you that we always have to anonymize the situation and the patient when writing the reflection note. It is quite possible to write a good reflection even if no personal information is included in the reflection note. We illustrate this way of working by using the story about Anna that we presented in Chapter 3. Note that the nurse dares to stand or stay in this conversation without having to know what Anna's life pain really is about until much farther along in the dialogue. By the nurse listening and asking open questions, Anna gains room and space to put into words what is important to her. Through this brief conversation, the nurse gains enough information to suggest that Anna can receive good help while still at the hospital.

ACTIVITY FOR INTERNAL REFLECTION AND DIALOGUE

Doing this reflective exercise on paper is very helpful when you first begin to practice reflexivity in nursing practice. Over time, you can begin to think about your attitude, words, and actions more deeply even without the written reflection. We do encourage you to keep on writing and analyzing your thoughts, words, and actions so that you keep on growing.

Box 4.1   Activity for Inner Dialogue

The conversation between *Anna* and the *nurse*	Internal reflection/dialogue of the *nurse*
	During the morning shift, I see that tears run down *Anna's* cheeks, but she smiles. . . Hmm, what is this? Is it just clearing her tear ducts? Or does something more lie behind the tears? How sad. . . I have taken a professional decision that, as far as possible, I should investigate what lies behind it when I get this unclear sense that I have just now, so I do well to explore the feeling a bit more.
Nurse: *Anna*, I see that you smile, but tears run down your cheeks. . .	I will describe what I see and see what happens. . .
Anna: I always smile – I have learned it. But inside me, I cry all the time.	I find that *Anna* opens up for something, but I still do not know what it is about. I venture to explore a little further, but notice that I must be careful.
Nurse: *Anna*, would you allow me to ask you a bit more about this?	Now I concentrate on being attentively present to *Anna*. She looks at me. The tears are running down her cheeks. I reach a hand out to her. I take care to signal to her that I listen attentively and see that she is vulnerable. *Anna* accepts my hand and I sit down beside her. This will show that I take my time.

The conversation between *Anna* and the *nurse*	Internal reflection/dialogue of the *nurse*
Anna: Yeah, that's fine.	I have gotten permission to go deeper. . .very gently.
Nurse: Would you like to tell a little bit more about what you are feeling and how things are for you right now?	I try to probe gently and hope the question is open enough for her to choose to walk the road further.
Anna: I have a large lump inside me that lies and weighs heavily.	I listen and suspect a deep pain at her heart.
I grew up in a Christian family, but my father was so strict and treated us badly. Therefore, I have not had anything to do with Christianity since I was young.	I listen and feel touched by the story.

Now, I see that she feels a little powerless. |
| Some years ago, we moved from the city to the countryside here. Because I have been so sick, I do not come out and do not have any contact with anyone other than home care nurses who came to us two weeks in the wake of my diagnosis. | What is it? Do I have anything more to contribute more here than an attentive presence?

I will be quiet and just listen. . . I squeeze her hand a little to show that I hear. |
| I have not told anyone about how things were in my childhood, so my husband does not know anything about this or how I feel now. | I suspect a kind of existential pain, but what is it?

I keep eye contact with *Anna* and hold her hand, and I will use silence. . . |

(Continued)

Box 4.1   (Continued)

The conversation between *Anna* and the *nurse*	Internal reflection/dialogue of the *nurse*
I have managed to hold on to this turmoil for many years, but now this pain inside me has become so big that I am unable to handle it anymore!	I wonder how she has been here for 12 days without finding anyone to talk to about this! Hmm, what do I say now? No easy answers. . .
In the ambulance on the way to the hospital, I asked God that I had to get to this hospital and that I had to get help, because it has become completely intolerable for me.	*Anna* said that she has a Christian background, but has distanced herself from it, but that she prayed to God in the ambulance. I need to know more about this before we can talk about how to get follow-up. What and who have been important for her through life? Who is she turning to when she needs help? I need to clarify. . .
Nurse: *Anna*, you say you grew up in a Christian home, but that you have distanced yourself from all that. Do you have anything that helps you with troubles now?	I keep holding *Anna's* hand to let her know I am fully here. I look at her face to listen as she answers and to think. . .
Anna: Yes, I have distanced myself from everything, but I have experienced many times in my life that God has been near and has helped me concretely. And I have a little hope that it can happen again. . .	I listen to the story and register that *Anna* describes a godly relationship and experience of God's presence in her life. The patient has been very open about the pain she knows and I feel she needs much more follow-up than I have time and the opportunity to give.

The conversation between Anna and the nurse	Internal reflection/dialogue of the nurse
	The conversation has taken less than 10 minutes and we are in the middle of the morning. I have to do rounds soon and will move on to the other patients under my care.
Nurse: *Anna*, I think you are very brave to tell me about what is so difficult for you. As you know, you have benefited from the treatment here and you will soon be discharged and going home to your husband. The time is short, so I suggest that you can talk more about this with a competent person on our staff.	I would do well to ask if the hospital chaplain can be a current conversation partner for the patient. . .

I will try to make sure that other groups in the hospital can contribute and will introduce the hospital chaplain's competence to go further with her, if she thinks it is possible to do so. |
My experience is that our hospital chaplains are good and wise conversation partners, and they have more time than nurses have here on the unit.	I try to convey that the chaplain is a safe person to open up to about deeply personal things.
If you think it is okay, I will contact you this morning so he can come to you today.	I ask permission so that it is not my decision but hers.
Anna: Yes, it's okay, you can do it.	Because I know that I myself do not have the ability to follow up as much as I would need to, I know very well that she can have follow-up with the hospital chaplain.
Nurse: That's good; then I will contact him soon so that he can start a conversation with you today.	Then I have secured that someone who will follow up and I have full confidence that our hospital chaplain will be able to help *Anna* in the best possible way.

Note: Exercise originally provided in NyNorsk in *Ondilig Omsorg* (Giske and Cone 2019).

Reflection 4.4

- Do you see the difficult points for the nurse in this conversation with Anna?
- What was it that made it difficult for the nurse?
- What do you think of such a way of reflecting on what was said and done by Anna and by the nurse caring for her?
- Think of a situation where you recognized and followed up a patient in the spiritual area. Write it in the same way that we have done with the story about Anna – with the conversation in the left column and the reflections you made along the way in the right column.
- Where were the difficult points in your conversation?
- What choices did you make during your nurse-patient talk?
- Were you able to think about what you were doing? Or have you had a chance to think about that interaction after the event?
- Is there anything from that reflection you want to bring into new situations?

FROM STORYTELLING TO CRITICAL REFLECTION

Telling about a situation simply gives a superficial and lower form of reflection, while a deeper reflection requires a repetitive process in which we use, summarize, and evaluate what has happened. One good way to learn such a systematic and deep reflection is to practice written reflection (Balgopal and Montplaisir 2011; Moon 2007; Sen 2010). Working with written reflections can be a safe way of working that makes it easier to be honest with the feelings and challenges we are familiar with in nursing practice. Our key points are important road signs in this process. Feelings of joy, of "getting it," of contact or connection, and that this was a meaningful or transcendent moment we interpret as being on the right path with what we do as nurses. Feelings of anger, frustration, and opposition or of doing any wrong can cause us to stop and become less passionate about integrating spirituality into practice. Reflection on those negative feelings can give us permission to change what we do or how we do it, in light of what we did, so that we can succeed and be more effective with our future actions in similar situations. It is important to reflect on the reasons we have for what we do because they can alert us so that we understand more about what is at stake in a given situation.

The writing process challenges us to create meaning in what happened by thinking about the mental and emotional state of the situation. When reflection requires us to ponder deeply, new meaning can emerge and we can discover new contexts in the experience because we draw on new perspectives and new knowledge. When we write down our reflections, we need to find our own words and concepts, which in turn stimulate the development of the professional language we have to help us grow as professionals (Balgopal and Montplaisir 2011).

Another aspect of writing a reflection note after the event is that in writing down our reflections, we must both think back to what has happened and we must think ahead to new and similar situations. The writer must also think about what was learned from past experience and knowledge that supports the assessment of the situation and that can justify future action choices. To gain the most help in developing nursing practice further, it is useful to be as specific and detailed as possible in terms of how we will follow up and change behavior from the discoveries we make in the work on the reflection notes (Sen 2010).

Below, we outline four points about the activity of examining and reflecting on a situation that can be helpful in written reflection work. By repeating this four-step pattern of writing things down, we can eventually learn to do the same work in our thoughts. This will then move the reflection process closer and closer to the actual action in the future as reflective actions become part of who we are as nurses.

Box 4.2 Activity for Reflection and Writing on Clinical Experiences

1. Write a brief note on the situation you want to reflect on. Note the time, place, the patient who was with you (use fictitious name), and explain what happened. Write down the thoughts and feelings you had in the situation as you thought and felt them.

2. Then write down your thinking about this situation afterwards.
   - What went well?
   - What contributed to what went well?
   - What happened just before the situation you are recalling?
   - What was your role in the situation?
   - If it did not look or feel very good, what was it that made you feel that way?

3. What can you learn from this situation that you can internalize and take with you so that the next time you experience something similar you can choose an even better way of acting? Write it down as clearly and concretely as possible.

   Is there something you need to learn more about or work with yourself on in relation to your thoughts, feelings, and actions? This point stimulates reflection on how we can become even better acquainted with ourselves and thus further develop our personal competence and get a more conscious relationship with the choice of action we can take with us into future situations.

4. To reach deeper reflection, it is also necessary to think about the knowledge you can gain as well as the understanding that can come from the situation. Consider various philosophical/theoretical perspectives, such as rapport building, meaning making, ethical theory, and more, to shed light on this; write down your inner dialogue.

Different theoretical perspectives can stimulate you to look at the situation from new angle. When it comes to spiritual care, relevant theories may be nursing theories that define some of our responsibilities, such as Travelbee's nursing theory on rapport building (McEwen and Wills 2017). Some of our work as nurses is based on the psychiatrist Victor Frankl's theory that the deepest human need is to experience meaning (Frankl 1946/1959). Ethical theory gives us guiding points to process ethical conflicts, and theories of communication address the complexity of verbal and nonverbal communication. We briefly presented Carl Jasper's theory of limit situations (Gatta 2015) in Chapter 1 as a framework for understanding what happens to people who experience different forms of loss. Drawing theory into reflection work and reflective practice is one way of systematically building professional identity and maturity. But remember that your deep reflection should be in your own words describing your inner thoughts.

Here is an example of what a reflection note can look like when using those four points for deep reflection that we have just gone through. The reflection note below is the work of a 1st year student who completed a required assignment to use Stoll's (1979) data collection guide (Chapter 2) in a practice encounter with someone who was not a patient. The student reflected on her conversation with another person.

1. Briefly describe the situation.
   I chose to talk to Maria (fictitious name), who is someone I know and is my own age. We talked about the four study guide questions: (1) foundation for hope and strength, (2) relationship between beliefs and health, (3) view of life and philosophy of life, and (4) faith and rituals or belief practices. The fourth point about a faith belief was not relevant since Maria had a humanistic view of life, and thus, no deity was addressed.

2. How I think about what happened.
   I think we had a good conversation, though I dreaded it at first when I saw that many of the questions are so personal.

Beginning with a reflection on hope and strength, Maria found these first and foremost from her family and friends, but she had great confidence in herself. Maria experienced it as hurtful to have people around who were fond of her and were afraid of losing hope and strength. She does not think that there is anything more than what we can understand with our senses, so her health beliefs have no transcendent element, and she feels that health is about good and right life choices. Since she has no faith in any concrete religion, worship means nothing to her. Maria did not think it would help to discuss this point, though she said that, if she *were* fascinated by the idea of faith, maybe it is something she would consider discussing in a crisis.

3. What I learned from the situation.

After the conversation, I have thought a lot about it because I myself have not thought through many of the questions we discussed. I feel that I see no clear relationship to whether I believe in anything specific. I feel unprepared to help patients in the spiritual area. I must admit that I feel anxiety and insecurity when I reflect on this theme. It is so hard for me, and it creates uncertainty. For me, it is almost taboo to think about growing old or getting ready to die. What happens afterwards? I cannot stand to think about it! I think that when I become a nurse, it is important to be able to show respect for the patient's thoughts, beliefs, and basis for hope and strength, even if it strives against my own thoughts on the subject. And I think that it is important for a conversation about this topic to happen at the patient's wishes. I am worried that I will not be able to become such an open nurse when I feel so uncertain and scared now. I hope that I will get help in my school classes and in practice over the next three years so that I can become more aware and be safer on this topic. This is important because we all have to decide our life-view since we are just here on earth for a short period. . .

4. Relevant theory to draw into the reflection.

   If I am going to choose a theory to reflect on after the conversation with Maria, then I think what we have learned about communication theory is relevant. When we try to map out the issues relating to personal spiritual needs and resources, the communication between the nurse and patient becomes their most important tool (Eide and Eide 2017). I have also read a research article where the nurses emphasized that it was important to follow the patient's language use and way of thinking (Ueland 2002). This is important, and I will become more aware of listening for it in conversations with patients when I am in clinical practice.

Reflection 4.5

- Think of a situation where you recognize and follow up on a patient in the spiritual area. Write a reflection note where you use the four points above.
- By doing this written reflection, did you discover anything new about the situation that can help you to grow personally and/or professionally?
- What theory is relevant to think about in the situation you chose? How did you apply the theory to your specific situation? What can you learn through that theory application?

ENDING UNFINISHED STORIES

We conclude this chapter with a storyline that shows that sometimes we may need help to enhance learning and to bring difficult experiences to a conclusion and integrate the learning into our own story and lifeview. If you have such unfinished experiences that you have not processed already, then we hope that this story can show you a way to work your way through that experience in a good way that can help you to gain perspective and to develop. It is possible to transform difficult and painful experiences into growth and wisdom (Hovland and Andresen 2007; Giske 2012).

We asked some healthcare professionals who retained a painful memory of patient situations after the patients went home, or the patient died, to share their thoughts. As we process the memory of one person, think of Figure 3.2 (Discerning the healing path), which we presented in Chapter 3. We do not suggest working through the whole three-stage process, even though it was obvious that the patient needed spiritual care. What we recommend is that you come to the memory with your personal antennae extended and already "tuned in" and that you work through the second phase to see what went on, then to think about what went well and what could have been done differently for a more positive outcome. There can be many reasons why the process breaks down, but knowing that one failed to help a patient who needed it can be an unfinished story in us. At a mindfulness conference, one nurse shared this story:

> We had a man, let us call him Marc, in our department. Marc was admitted with long-term cancer at end-stage of the disease. It had spread to the liver, and his skin was yellow and he had fluid in his abdomen. Marc attended a charismatic congregation and often had visits by both the family and people from the congregation. Marc was happy and excited because he was prayed for, and he thought he would become well. He had an anointed cloth under the pillow as a sign of this. Marc had received a Bible word as a promise from one of his church leaders: You will live and tell your children and grandchildren about the great work of God.
>
> Marc's condition became worse by the day, but it was not possible for us in the department to talk to either Marc or his family about him probably dying of his disease very shortly. Talking about death was "not faithful to God's promise" (according to them).

Marc was dying, and the family did not say good-bye or make any farewell gestures to him, so his death was a bad situation for everyone. Those working in that department were not very good at talking with each other either about deep things, so both along the way and afterwards, and many times since then, I have pondered on this painful experience, all without getting it out of my system.

One of the leaders at the conference asked if the nurse wanted help to work through this experience, so she said, "yes, thank you." Then they put an empty chair that represented the patient into the center of the circle of attendees, and they invited the nurse to picture the patient on the chair and tell the patient how she had experienced nursing him while he was ill and what she had wanted to say to him. The nurse did so, and everyone in the group listened. Afterwards, there was a time for reflection to tell what they thought the patient would have said if he could answer. Again, the nurse was invited to talk to the patient as if he had more on his heart than anyone had said, or if there was something different she thought the patient might have said. This work helped the nurse to complete the relationship with the patient and to bring closure for her. She could integrate the experience into her life with a greater courage to dare to talk about what was difficult both in relation to patients and families, as well as to colleagues. The others in attendance also learned from this activity.

Reflection 4.6

- What do you think about this "empty chair" type of exercise? Could it be helpful to you?
- Do you have for one or more such unfinished stories in relation to patients or relatives you have met? What is it about the situation that makes it an unfinished story?
- What have you done to try to create meaning and to clarify your role in what happened?
- Do you see ways you could get help to complete any of your unfinished stories?

REFLECTING ON WHAT YOU KNOW AND WHAT YOU NEED TO LEARN

We all change over time, and it is very important to recognize that this is a normal and even positive thing – it is growth, both personal and professional growth, that can help us become better people and more effective nurses. Intentional reflection can help us recognize the things that are influencing us to change, as well as the patterns that have developed in us from our background, our culture, our families, and more. Patterns may be good and positive, but they may also be problematic and negative. Reflection helps to understand ourselves better and to see what we need to learn or how we need to change. Reflecting through our personal journals or through assigned work, written or verbal, as individuals or in groups, is critical to our personal and professional growth (Cone and Giske 2018). Even skills can be improved through reflection!

SPIRITUAL CARE SKILLS AND COMPETENCIES

Dutch nursing scholars Rene van Leeuwen and Bart Cusveller (2004) were some of the first to research and write about the basic competence nurses should have in spiritual care upon completing a bachelor's degree in nursing. Presenting such competency standards for spiritual care to other nurse scholars led to a discussion as to how this can best be followed up in education and what focus it should have in practice, and thus the network of spiritual care scholars became formalized, and work on this Spiritual Care Education Standard became the focus of scholars across Europe and around the world (www.epicc-network.org). Initially, van Leeuwen and Cusveller developed three domains with a total of six core areas for spiritual care competence. We present the domains and competence areas in an overview to facilitate understanding of them:

Domain 1: Awareness and use of self
- Competence 1: Nurses handle their own values and beliefs and feelings in the professional relationship they have with patients with other faiths and other religions.

- Competence 2: The nurse addresses the subject of spirituality with patients from different cultures in a caring manner.

Domain 2: Spiritual dimensions of nursing
- Competence 3: The nurse collects information about the patient's spirituality and identifies the patient's need.
- Competence 4: The nurse discusses with patients and team members how spiritual care is planned, provided, and reported.
- Competence 5: The nurse provides spiritual care and evaluates it with the patient and team members.

Domain 3: Assurance of quality and expertise
- Competence 6: The nurse contributes to quality assurance and to improving expertise in spiritual care.

These six areas of expertise are a good starting point for discussing how nursing education should build up teaching in order to ensure that students develop a reflective relationship with their own beliefs and property within three years. We have given many ideas on how to prepare both nurse and the student in Chapter 2. One area we did not yet emphasize is the "art of the oral hand-off" (Giske et al. 2018), which is an important skill alluded to in the second domain with both competencies 4 and 5 as well as in competency 6 within the third domain.

The first competence points to an important relationship that may sometimes be difficult to know how one should relate to. How are we going to handle our self-esteem and convictions when we meet patients who have a completely different view of life than us? It may be that the one party has a religious outlook and the other does not, or that one has different religious beliefs. Facilitating special food and other practical concerns for patients with a different outlook should not be difficult for anyone. Problems usually occur when we do not know when it is okay to read religious texts to a patient if we are not religious ourselves or when we do not share the patient's faith. It may even be more personal and thus more difficult if a patient asks us to pray, when we do not share the patient's beliefs. Please take a moment to reflect on the following questions.

Reflection 4.7

- Will the boundaries between what is of help to the patient and what I as a nurse know are okay for me to participate in be crossed?

- Am I, as a nurse, allowed to say no to what a patient is asking me to do?

- What type of spiritual care can I provide that would be most helpful to the patient?

This is when teamwork on a unit can be especially helpful. When a team knows the skills, beliefs, and comfort level with the spiritual domain, then members can call on each other for specific situations; hopefully, the chaplain is an integrated member of the healthcare team, which makes referrals more easily done (Giske and Cone 2015).

Norwegian regulations on the common framework plan for health and social studies say that after completing bachelor education, the candidate must contribute to ensuring equal services for all groups in our society, regardless of age and gender, ethnicity, religion, and vision, etc (Forskrift, 2017, p. 2.2). We understand this as a clear expectation that the nurse will be able to make sure that patients receive the spiritual care they want. This is also in line with the ethical code of the International Council of Nurses (2021), which says that nurses should seek to create a climate in which patients and their families will feel that values, customs and beliefs are respected. The circular from the Norwegian Ministry of Health and Care Services (2009) emphasizes the same, namely that those who receive municipal health and care services, which in Norway are part of the city government's responsibility, have the right to exercise their own values and life-views. The right to exercise an individual's view of life is seen as one of the basic needs, and thus part of the health and care concept.

Students sometimes tell stories from home-based practices where data collection among patients with dementia shows that earlier in life they had the habit of praying an evening prayer or an "Our Father" when they went to sleep. An example is where an evening prayer was hung over the bed of a patient so that everyone could easily follow this up. Then it turned out that the note about evening prayers was taken down by the staff because they did not share the patient's faith or believe in prayer (Kuven and Bjørvatn, 2015). Our view is that when such challenges come up in practice, then it is the nurse's responsibility to find ways to ensure that the individual patient gets the spiritual care they need (Cockell and McSherry 2012). The individual student and nurse must also reflect and work with themselves to understand more of why this is so difficult and what it means to be professional. The nursing team one works with must discuss how to jointly plan nursing care so that when it is important to the patients to be able to read an evening prayer, then someone on the team can do so.

For some patients, it may be enough that we offer fellowship with them by making eye contact and listening to what the patient is asking (Koenig 2013; Taylor 2007). For those who have different ways of thinking or some form of cognitive impairment and cannot follow personal practices for themselves anymore, one should be able to be flexible to provide spiritual care at the patient's level. Nurses have experienced that just reading a familiar poem or sacred literature or prayer to a patient with dementia can be comforting. One woman had done this as a regular evening ritual together with her husband for their entire life together. It was good to see how, in spite of her current dementia, this well-known prayer was what she needed to comfort her in the evening and to settle her down to sleep without the need for sleeping medication.

If we look further at domain 2 and competencies 3–5 presented by van Leeuwen and Cusveller (2013), we see that these are about what happens from data collection to assessment, planning in the team, implementation, and reporting. These are processes we wrote about in Chapter 3. However, we have some comments about this domain. Firstly, we believe that it is important that students and nurses are open to the fact that spiritual concerns can be important for patients, but that it is not always a comfortable topic for health personnel. In the same way that not all patients have problems with circulation or respiration, it is not always the case that spiritual/existential concerns are important for all patients. This means that we have to be open to the fact that it may or may not be relevant, but that in a specific situation we must do a professional assessment of what is important for this patient. To be able to do such an assessment, we strongly recommend that the nurse develop different questions to ask that give the patient an opportunity for them to open up and reveal what is relevant for them. We have shown various open questions that can be used both in Chapters 2 and 3.

The other aspect we would like to comment on is that in competence 3, van Leeuwen and Cusveller (2013) say that it is the patients' spiritual needs that must be identified. This is very true, but we also believe that it is very important to identify patients' spiritual resources. Having a narrow focus just on needs gives us an inaccurate picture of the person. Research in spirituality and health (Koenig et al. 2012) shows that religious support is a major factor in improving health outcomes for patients. In the spiritual arena, it is important that we understand what resources give hope and meaning to patients or provide connection, love, and belonging to them. Once we understand what resources they have, we can help them to access these resources.

The last comment we have about van Leeuwen and Cusveller (2013) is related to the sixth competence – that students and nurses are not supposed to have a personal agenda when it comes to the quality of spiritual care. Students and nurses have a responsibility to develop the quality of spiritual care in the team, in the unit, and in the organization where we work. Development of quality in the provision of spiritual care must be an integral part of nursing education, which is the responsibility of clinical supervisors and educators in the workplace just as we continuously evaluate quality of nutrition and hygiene and other aspects of patient care (Cone and Giske 2018). The standard for spiritual care must also be visible in professional guidelines.

Reflection 4.8

- Do you think that the patient has the right to exercise his or her own view of life as part of healthcare services?
- What contradictions do you see between the patient's rights and your duty when patients have a different outlook on life than you?
  - If you have seen this, how did you solve it?
  - How did you justify your choice professionally?

FEATURES AND QUALIFICATIONS OF THE HELPER

In Norway's national guidelines for palliative care among cancer patients, one section address qualities and qualifications that are important in facilitating spiritual care (Norwegian Directorate of Health 2015). These guidelines do not focus on what new nurses should be able to do to complete their education, but rather, they point out what patients in palliative or end-of-life care should be able to expect from encounters with healthcare personnel. However, we can consider different patient populations because these guidelines can apply to anyone who is in the vulnerable position of a patient, and students and nurses may experience challenges in the face of the seriously ill, the debilitated, and patients in deep suffering. Spiritual care is a responsibility of the entire team, but it is as individuals that we meet patients, assess situations, and follow up on the individual patient issue (Giske 2012). These guidelines point to the need for us to continuously work with ourselves in these areas in order to provide whole person care to patients. Moreover, these principles apply globally and are acknowledged as important concerns in most nursing textbooks, especially those with a chapter on spirituality and spiritual care as is true in the USA.

Here are the points that the guidelines emphasize as important attributes and qualifications of health professionals:

- the ability to feel empathy and sympathy in the different aspects of human life and people's differences
- a relationship with one's own spirituality, faith, and beliefs of life and death
- one's own motivation to think holistically about the situation of the seriously ill and the dying, and the ability to detect and respond adequately to spiritual issues
- the ability to pay attention to and have respect for patients' own efforts toward spiritual maturity
- knowledge of the spiritual area and how serious illness and death influence spirituality
- the ability to listen and to be fully present, even in situations where one feels helpless and powerless
- the ability to understand and communicate in ways that combine honesty and sensitivity
- an ability to live with unresolved questions, both by themselves and with the patient
- the ability to utilize guidance and "debriefing" with peers and supervisors
- an ability to set aside oneself and one's own problems and solutions in order to accommodate the other. (NDH 2015, p. 35)

It may seem very difficult to be accept feeling helpless and powerless and still be able to live with unresolved questions in the face of serious illness and death. Being able to put our own problems aside to make room for the other person can also be quite challenging. We support this way of thinking about nursing, especially when meeting people in vulnerable situations. Being able to accept that we cannot fix everything challenges us to meet people where they are and "just" be there with them (Carson, 2011). The Danish theologian and philosopher Løgstrup (2020) wrote that it is part of our basic condition as human beings that we are dependent on others. He explains that we are "aliens" in this world, and we often meet situations where we cannot relate to another person without being completely vulnerable to them. Løgstrup explains his perspective in a way that relates to nursing. The qualities and qualifications the nurse must have when we have such a great responsibility for other people's lives include both the small and large moments that are important to the other, so the patient is completely vulnerable to the nurse, and in some ways, nurses are vulnerable to our patients when we open ourselves up to walk their journey with them. So, whether the patient lives or dies, recovers or maintains life in a new way with a chronic illness, what we nurses say and do is critically important.

In order to develop these traits, it is helpful to learn how to reflect deeply both alone and together with others. As nurse educators and leaders, it is very important that we give room for students and nurses to have dialogue where our experiences, feelings, and thoughts can be brought into focus. Without such safe spaces, it is impossible to stand and face all the challenges of life. Educators must take on the responsibility for creating these spaces on behalf of our students in nursing programs. For students and nurses working in clinical practice, it is a responsibility of the team manager or the unit leader, who must take seriously the need to create a welcoming work environment (Cockell and McSherry 2012).

Reflection 4.9

- Have you felt helpless and powerless in the face of patient's needs? What do you do when you feel this way?
- To what extent are you able to set your own problems and solutions aside to accommodate the patient?
- What do you need from the working community to be able to listen and be present for patients?

MOVING FROM STUDENT TO NURSE

The three middle chapters of this handbook are based on a learning spiral model for spiritual care that is an iterative three-phased spiral of learning through education and professional practice. First, we prepare ourselves by seeking new insights and knowledge about ourselves, our own spirituality, and our responsibility for competency in spiritual care (Chapter 2). Then as we connect with patients, we apply our new knowledge in practice where we recognize, and follow up different patients in the spiritual area with openness, honesty, and courage (Chapter 3). Finally, we reflect on these experiences, on what was well done and what was not so well done, which can then be transformed into new life experiences, growth, and wisdom through our reflections, both individually and in groups (Chapter 4).

Personal and professional growth is a learning spiral that repeats throughout life as we seek and gain new knowledge about ourselves and others (Chapter 5). In 2002, McSherry and Ross wrote that in nursing practice we will often face things that are deeply important to patients but that are dilemmas for us as nurses. This is still true today. Students and nurses need to continue to develop greater understanding and competencies in spiritual care over their life and professional practice. Because each person we serve is unique and each situation is different, we are never fully trained in this area, so the learning spiral keeps on going in a lifelong cycle as we prepare for more encounters, connect with patients, and reflect on our attitudes and actions related to spiritual care. This learning spiral is rather like a helix that expands ever onward and helps the nurse to grow personally and professionally throughout life (Cone and Giske 2013a). We can assess our personal growth in spiritual care through the Spiritual Care Competency Self-Assessment Tool (see the EPICC website: www.epicc-network.org) that is presented in the next chapter. In addition to addressing the importance of lifelong learning in the final chapter, we also present ways for nurses to take care of ourselves to avoid burnout, develop coping strategies, encourage kindness and civility, learn assertiveness, and mitigate bullying, as well as to create a welcoming and healing environment wherever we serve. Spiritual care is thus presented as important for both the patient, through our nurse-patient interactions, and the nurse, through spiritual self-care.

REFERENCES

Balgopal, M.M. and Montplaisir, L.M. (2011). Meaning making: what reflective essays reveal about biology students' concepts about natural selection. *Instructional Science* 39: 137–169. https://doi.org/10.1007/s11251-009-9120-y.

Carson,V. B. (2011). What is the essence of spiritual care? *Journal of Christian Nursing* 28 (3): 173.

Cockell, N. and McSherry, W. (2012). Spiritual care in nursing: an overview of published international research. *Journal of Nursing Management* 20 (8): 958–969. https://doi.org/10.1111/j.1365-2834.2012.01450.x.

Cone, P.H. (2016). Commentary on the importance of spiritual literacy. *Christian Nurses International: Partnerships (A Journal of NCFI)* 1 (7): 17–19.

Cone, P.H. and Giske, T. (2013a). Open journey theory – intersection of journeying with students and opening up to learning spiritual care. *Journal of Nursing Education and Practice* 3 (11): 1–9.

Cone, P.H. and Giske, T. (2017). Nurses' comfort level with spiritual assessment: a mixed method study among nurses working in diverse healthcare settings. *Journal of Clinical Nursing* 26 (19–20): 3125–3136. https://doi.org/10.1111/jocn.13660.

Cone, P.H. and Giske, T. (2018). Integrating spiritual care into nursing education and practice: strategies utilizing open journey theory. *Journal of Nurse Education Today* 71: 22–25.

Eide, H. and Eide, T. (2017). *Kommunikasjon i relasjoner. Personorientering, samhandling, etikk*, 3e. *Communication in Relationships: Person Orientation, Interaction, Ethics*. Gyldendal Akademiske.

Forskrift om felles rammeplan for helse- og sosialfagutdanninger(2017). https://lovdata.no/dokument/SF/forskrift/2017-09-06-1353

Frankl, V. (1946/1959). *Man's Search for Meaning. [Tr from German by Ilse Lasch]*. Beacon Press.

Gatta, G. (2015). Suffering and the making of politics: Perspectives from Jaspers and Camus. *Contemporary Political Theory* 14 (4): 335–354.

Giske, T. (2012). How undergraduate nursing students learn spiritual care in clinical studies – a review of literature. *Journal of Nursing Management* 20: 1049–1057.

Giske, T. and Cone, P.H. (2012). Opening up for learning: a grounded theory study of nursing student education on spiritual care. *Journal of Clinical Nursing* 21 (13–14): 2006–2015.

Giske, T. and Cone, P.H. (2015). Discerning the healing path: how nurses assist patients spiritually in diverse healthcare settings. *Journal of Clinical Nursing* 24: 10–20. 10.111/jocn.12907.

Giske, T. and Cone, P.H. (2019). *Å ta vare på heile mennesket: Handbok i åndeleg omsorg [Caring for the Whole Person: Handbook of Spiritual Care]*. Samlaget.

Giske, T., Melås, S.N., and Einarsen, K.A. (2018). The art of oral handover: a participant observational study by undergraduate students in a hospital setting. *Journal of Critical Nursing* 27 (5–6): e767–e775. https://doi.org/10.1111/jocn.14177.

Giske, T., Schep-Akkerman, A., Bø, B., Cone, P. H., Moene Kuven, B., Mcsherry, W., Owasu, B., Ueland, V., Lassche-Scheffer, J., van Leeuwen, R., & Ross, L. (2022). Developing and testing the EPICC Spiritual Care Competency Self-Assessment Tool for student nurses and midwives. *Journal of Clinical Nursing*.

Hovland, O.J. and Andresen, G.S. (2007). Integrering i praksisfellesskapet med refleksjon som verktøy [Integration into the community of practice with reflection as a tool]. In: *Engasjement Og læring. Fagkritiske Perspektiv på Sykepleie [Commitment and Learning: Professionally Critical Perspectives on Nursing]* (ed. H. Alvsvåg and O. Førland), 189–203. Akribe.

International Council of Nurses [ICN] (2021). ICN Code of Ethics for Nurses. https://www.icn.ch/system/files/2021-10/ICN_Code-of-Ethics_EN_Web_0.pdf (accessed 22 March 2022).

Koenig, H.G. (2013). *Spirituality in Patient Care: Why, How, When, and What*, 3ee. Templeton Press https://doi.org/10.1177/0898010115580236.

Koenig, H.G., King, D., and Carson, V.B. (2012). *Handbook in Religion and Health*. Oxford University Press.

Kuven, B. M., & Bjørvatn, L. (2015). Spiritual care: part of nursing? *Christian Nurse International* 5: 4–8.

Løgstrup, K.E. (2020). *The Ethical Demand*. Oxford University Press. [Originally in Danish (1956) from Gyldendal.]

McEwen, M. and Wills, E.M. (2017). *Theoretical Frameworks for Nursing*, 5ee. Lippincott Williams & Wilkens.

Molander, B. (2015). *The Practice of Knowing and Knowing in Practice*. Peter Lang. [Originally in Swedish (1996) from Daidalos.]

Moon, J. (2007). Getting the measure of reflection: considering matters of definition and depth. *Journal of Radiotherapy in Practice* 6 (4): 191–200. https://doi.org/10.1017/S1460396907006188.

Neathery, M., Taylor, E. J., & He, Z. (2020b). Perceived barriers to providing spiritual care among psychiatric mental health nurses. *Archives of Psychiatric Nursing* 34 (6): 572–579. https://doi.org/10.1016/j.apnu.2020.10.004.

Norwegian Directorate of Health [NDH] (2015). National guidelines for handling patients in palliative care [Helsedirektoratet: Nasjonalt handlingsprogram for palliasjon i kreftomsorgen]. IS-2285. NMHCS, Oslo.

Norwegian Ministry of Health and Care Services [NMHC] (2009). *Opptrappingsplan for psykisk helse 1999–2006*. [Step-up plan for mental health services 1999–2006].

Oslo University Hospital (2018). [Oslo Universitetssykehus] *Helsepersonells roller i åndelig og eksistensiell omsorg i møte med pasienter* [Healthcare professionals' roles in meeting patients' spiritual and existential care]. https://ehandboken.ous-hf.no/document/134012#23 (accessed 5 December 2021).

Ross, L., McSherry, W., van Leeuwen, R. et al. (2018). Nursing and midwifery students' perceptions of spirituality, spiritual care, and spiritual care competency: a prospective, longitudinal, correlational European study. *Nurse Education Today* 24–71. https://doi.org/10.1016/j.nedt.2018.05.002.

Rykkje, L.R., Eriksson, K., and Råholm, M.B. (2013). Spirituality and caring in old age and the significance of religion: A hermeneutical study from Norway. *Scandinavian Journal of Caring Science* 27: 275–284. https://doi.org/10.1111/j.1471-6712.2012.01028.x.

Schön, D. (1983/2001) *The Reflective Practitioner: How Professionals Think in Action.* Basic Books.

Sen, B.A. (2010). Reflective writing: a management skill. *Library Management* 31 (1/2): 79–93. https://doi.org/10.1108/01435121011013421.

Stoll, R.I. (1979). Guidelines for spiritual assessment. *American Journal of Nursing* 79 (9): 1572–1577.

Taylor, E.J. (2007). *What Do I Say? Talking with Patients about Spirituality.* Templeton Foundation Press.

Ueland, V. (2002). Sykepleieren og den åndelige/eksistensielle samtalen. Hvordan kan vi konkret samtale med pasienten? [the nurse and the spiritual/existential conversation. How can we concretely talk with the patient?]. *Kreftsykepleie [Cancer Nursing]* 3: 11–19.

van Leeuwen, R. and Cusveller, B. (2004). Nursing competencies for spiritual care. *Journal of Advance Nursing* 48 (3): 234–245. https://doi.org/10.1111/j.1365-2648.2004.03192.x.

van Leeuwen, R. and Cusveller, B. (2013). Nursing competencies for spiritual care. *Journal of Advanced Nursing* 48 (3): 234–246. https://doi.org/10.1111/j.1365-2648.2004.03192.x.

CHAPTER 5

Lifelong Learning, Self-Care, and Workplace Care

Every nurse needs to focus on being a lifelong learner, each of us taking care of our own self for the good of all. In this final chapter, we discuss a variety of resources to help nurses care for yourselves, manage stress, avoid burnout, and promote a welcoming and healing environment so that you remain healthy and balanced and thrive as a nurse in a constantly changing world. We discuss the current state of healthcare in the world, especially in the USA, where bullying is a serious issue and the workplace environment can be hostile instead of welcoming. We encourage all nurses to hold a "no tolerance" policy for such negative behaviors. Let us all be difference makers and change agents so that we can promote a healthy and hospitable environment where patient care naturally includes the spiritual domain as part of holistic nursing care and where the importance of promoting a welcoming environment for all healthcare professionals in the workplace is clear. As we conclude our handbook, we encourage both working nurses and

The Nurse's Handbook of Spiritual Care, First Edition. Pamela Cone and Tove Giske.
© 2022 John Wiley & Sons Ltd. Published 2022 by John Wiley & Sons Ltd.

nursing students to continue learning about spirituality and spiritual care – it truly is a lifelong thing. . .

LIFELONG LEARNING

World-renowned nurse philosopher and theorist Patricia Benner has emphasized the importance of building on knowledge and experience with her *Novice to Expert Model* (Benner 1984). The focus of her model is learning and growing into our professional role as nurses, from the first moment we enter a nursing program through the years of study and then practical experience until we become expert nurses (Alligood 2018; McEwen and Wills 2017). Benner shows us, moreover, that there is always more to learn no matter how expert we become in any particular area (Figure 5.1). For example, one may be truly expert in understanding the Christian world view but a novice with other world religions or with the humanistic perspective. Her model is a reminder that we need to keep growing and learning. This idea is highlighted in the book *Critical Reflection, Spirituality and Professional Practice* by Cheryl Hunt, where she discusses how our life is a journey, a road through our landscape/environment, as we "journey on a long and winding road passing through a rich, variegated landscape"(2021, p. 185) shaped by our personal worldview.

Benner describes five levels of learning: (1) Novice (new/no experience/rule-governed), (2) Advanced Beginner (has some experience/principle-based judgment), (3) Competent (has a few years of experience/actions based on consensus, analysis), (4) Proficient (has much experience/learns and modifies based on situations), and (5) Expert (very experienced/intuitive, flexible, highly proficient). To develop more expertise in spiritual care, we turn to the work of our European colleagues and the EPICC (**E**nhancing nurses' and midwives' competence in **P**roviding spiritual care through **I**nnovative education and **C**ompassionate **C**are) Network of spiritual care scholars that has been doing research and writing on this domain for over 20 years (www.epicc-network.org).

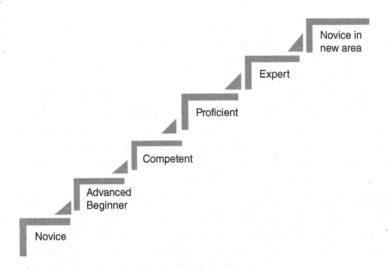

FIGURE 5.1   The Nurse is always learning – Benner's Novice to Expert Model (1984). *Source*: *Note: Adapted from the work of Benner (1984).

SPIRITUAL CARE EDUCATIONAL STANDARD FOR NURSING COMPETENCY IN SPIRITUAL CARE

The initial work on spiritual care competencies of Dutch scholar Dr. Rene van Leeuwen (van Leeuwen and Cusveller 2004) and that of Dr. Josephine Attard from Malta was the foundation for a bachelor standard of education in spiritual care. The work of these scholars was the springboard for a large European network of spiritual care research scholars and teachers from various bachelor's degree in nursing and midwifery programs who worked together to further develop (Attard et al. 2019a, 2019b; van Leeuwen et al. 2009) a common European standard of spiritual care competencies (EPICC Project: www.epicc-network.org). that are free to all. Norwegian nurse scholars like the second author have been part of the EPICC Network, and California scholars, including the first author, later joined this network, believing that this sound work in spiritual care is appropriate for nurses around the world. Upon completion of a bachelor-level degree, healthcare professionals in all fields should have competencies in a variety of areas, including spiritual care competencies, though nurses and midwives are the primary focus of the EPICC Network (van Leeuwen et al. 2020).

Student perspectives were explored for different formulations and competency areas in 8 different countries in Europe (Ross et al. 2018). A three-year process, where nursing and midwifery scholars and educators from 21 countries in Europe explored and developed four areas of spiritual competencies (van Leeuwen et al. 2020), resulted in the Network proposing four areas of spiritual care as common to European nursing education and focused on knowledge, skills, and attitudes related to each competency area. All materials are now housed and freely available on the website at the University of Staffordshire in England, UK (www.epicc-network.org). The EPICC Network believes that nurses, midwives, and educators should help nursing and midwifery students and working nurses globally to grow in the areas of intra-personal spirituality, inter-personal spirituality, assessment and planning of spiritual care, and intervention and evaluation of spiritual care. These four elements are described below:

1. **Intrapersonal Spirituality:** The student is aware of the importance of spirituality for health and well-being. This area of expertise is about recognizing the importance of the spirit of a person in relation to health and well-being. The student should understand the concept of spirituality and be able to explain how the spirit affects health and well-being throughout their life. Students must be able to understand how their own values and beliefs influence the exercise of spiritual care among patients and be able to reflect on and recognize that there can be differences based on patients' beliefs and values. The students also need to be able to care for themselves and be willing to explore patients' personal, religious, and spiritual beliefs and be open to and respectful of the person's multiple expressions of spirituality.

2. **Interpersonal Spirituality:** Students engage in the patient/client/family's spirituality, and recognize the unique spiritual and cultural outlook, beliefs, and practices. This area of expertise is about understanding how people express their spirituality. In this area of competence, it is important to know the different ways deep inner beliefs and/or religious views can influence how people react to important life events. The student should be able to recognize the unique nature of each person's spirituality. Furthermore, the student should collaborate with the person and exercise spiritual care with sensitivity and genuine caring. It is important that students build confidence and are easy to approach and that they act respectfully in the face of another person's expressions of spirituality and various beliefs and practices.

3. **Spiritual Care: Assessment and Planning:** The student considers spiritual needs and resources using customized formal or informal ways to collect data and plan spiritual care, maintain confidentiality, and get informed consent when needed. This area of competence is about student understanding of what spiritual care is and knowing different ways to collect data and to make a spiritual assessment. The student should also know the role of other professionals, such as chaplains and special counselors, in exercising spiritual care. The student should have an open and non-judgmental attitude and be willing and able to accommodate and handle feelings that arise during a spiritual encounter.

4. **Spiritual Care: Intervention and Evaluation:** Students act in relation to spiritual needs and resources in a caring and compassionate manner. The last area of expertise is that the student nurse is aware of the significance of compassion and presence in spiritual care and knows how to identify needs and resources in an appropriate manner so that needs can be addressed. The student should also be able to assess whether spiritual needs have been met, so that this area is no longer where to focus nursing care. Furthermore, a student must recognize personal boundaries in spiritual care and balance them with professional

boundaries. Nursing students need to be able to refer their patients to other healthcare professionals as needed. For example, teamwork with chaplains is of critical importance in spirituality (Giske and Cone 2015).

After a spiritual care intervention, the student should also be able to evaluate and document personal, professional, and organizational conditions for exercising spiritual care and be able to reassess and modify the plan as needed. The student who is welcoming and accepting and demonstrates empathy, open heartedness, professional kindness and love in collaborating with others and, if necessary, seeking spiritual support from others will be able to integrate the spiritual naturally into whole person, patient-centered care. Furthermore, the student should be able to carry out and document spiritual care in a respectful and non-judgmental manner; this includes being able to cooperate with other professionals and make referrals as needed. The Spiritual Care Competency Educational Standard developed by the EPICC Network is shown in Reflection 5.1.

Reflection 5.1

- Review the four areas of competencies and reflect on your personal competencies; assess your own competence on a scale from 1–5 where 1 is least and 5 is most.
- Go to the EPICC website (www.epicc-network.org); a Spiritual Care Competencies Self-Assessment Tool is now available for free use globally.
- In what area did you do well and what area do you need to develop further?

TIPS FOR NURSING EDUCATORS

Whether you are a nurse or nursing student, everything we have addressed applies in some way to all levels of nursing. Actually, professional nurses, nursing students, and nurse educators all need to participate in lifelong learning. Educators can use an

Box 5.1 EPICC Spiritual Care Competencies Standard for BSNs

Competencies	Knowledge (Cognition)	Skills (Function)	Attitude (Affect) ((Affective) (Behavioral)
1. Intrapersonal Spirituality: Is aware of the importance of spirituality on health and well-being.	• Understands the concept of spirituality. • Can explain the impact of spirituality on a person's health and well-being across the lifespan for oneself and others. • Understands the impact of one's own values and beliefs in providing spiritual care.	• Reflects meaningfully upon one's own values and beliefs and recognizes that these may be different from other people. • Takes care of oneself.	• Willing to explore one's own and individuals' personal, religious and spiritual beliefs. • Is open and respectful to people's diverse expressions of spirituality.
2. Interpersonal Spirituality:	• Understands the ways that people express their spirituality.	• Recognizes the uniqueness of people's spirituality.	• Is trustworthy, approachable and respectful of people's expressions of spirituality and different world/religious views.

(*Continued*)

Box 5.1 (Continued)

Competencies	Knowledge (Cognition)	Skills (Function)	Attitude (Affect) ((Affective) (Behavioral)
Engages with people's spirituality, acknowledging their unique spiritual and cultural worldviews, beliefs, and practices.	• Is aware of the different world/religious views and how these may impact upon people's responses to key life events.	• Interacts with, and responds sensitively to the person's spirituality.	
3. Spiritual Care: Assessment/Planning: Assesses spiritual needs and resources using appropriate formal or informal approaches, and plans spiritual care, maintains patient confidentiality, obtains informed consent.	• Understands the concept of spiritual care. • Is aware of different approaches to spiritual assessment. • Understands other professionals' roles in providing spiritual care.	• Conducts and documents a spiritual assessment to identify spiritual needs and resources. • Collaborates with other professionals. • Be able to appropriately contain and deal with emotions.	• Is open, approachable and non-judgmental. • Has a willingness to deal with emotions.

Spiritual Care: Intervention and Evaluation: Responds to spiritual needs and resources within a caring, compassionate relationship.	• Understands the concept of compassion and presence and its importance in spiritual care. • Knows how to respond appropriately to identified spiritual needs and resources. • Knows how to evaluate whether spiritual needs have been met.	• Recognizes personal limitations in spiritual care giving and refers to others as appropriate. • Evaluates and documents personal, professional and organizational aspects of spiritual care giving, and reassess appropriately.	• Shows compassion and presence. • Shows willingness to collaborate with and refer to others (professional/ non- professional). • Is welcoming and accepting and shows empathy, openness, professional humility and trustworthiness in seeking additional spiritual support.

integrative strategy to create a threaded learning experience across the nursing curriculum that avoids adding courses to an already heavy learning program (Cone 2020; Rykkje et al. 2021; Taylor et al. 2014). Real patient scenarios are useful to help students work through what they might say in a given situation, so they should be tailored to whatever learning module is currently being taught (Cone and Giske 2018; Taylor et al. 2014). There are many useful strategies, including the use of simulation and live actors in role plays, for promoting learning among our nursing students. However, the most important thing is for educators to raise student awareness of the spiritual domain and to help them prepare for spirituality and its relationship to health, connect with patients at a deep level, and reflect on their encounters with patients, both what we felt went well and what did not go so well (Cone and Giske 2013b). This needs to be done at every level and in every course across the curriculum rather than simply adding in a Spiritual Care course to the nursing program.

One important thing to note is that for any student or nurse learning from a nursing educator, growth involves a gradual release of responsibility (GRR), depicted as a pair of reverse pyramids (Fisher and Frey 2013b). In this model, the teacher begins with explaining (broad base of upside-down 1st pyramid) and demonstrating concepts in focused lessons while the student (tip of 2nd pyramid) sits and listens. Guided instruction follows as the teacher and student begin to connect, such as when the teacher correctly places a stethoscope on a person's chest while the student listens for heart and/or breath sounds. The next stage of the GRR is collaborative as the student and teacher do it together with the student taking on a little more initiative for the work. Finally, the teacher relinquishes the primary role (1st pyramid tip) and the student works independently, having become more knowledgeable and is taking on the responsibility for learning (Fisher and Frey 2013a). This way of structured teaching is a little easier to carry out when there is a physical task to do, but role modeling compassionate care, active listening, engaged presence, and therapeutic communication that delves cautiously but courageously into what is deeply important to the patient is one of the best ways to help students learn how to facilitate spiritual care. Figure 5.2 shows another perspective on the

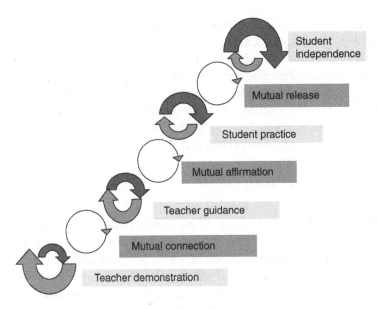

Student
independence

Mutual release

Student practice

Mutual affirmation

Teacher guidance

Mutual connection

Teacher demonstration

FIGURE 5.2   GRR (Gradual Release of Responsibility) adapted by Cone.

concept of teaching/learning. The lower arrow represents the teacher, who has more knowledge investment in the beginning, while the upper arrow stands for the student who has limited knowledge at first that grows as students learn more and take on more responsibility for the learning aspect of this mutual process.

   While it is critically important for nurses to keep learning and growing both personally and professionally, it is equally important that we take good care of ourselves so that we can thrive amidst the challenges of today (Hill and Smith 1990). This is, in fact, a moral and ethical mandate from the *Code of Ethics for Nurses with interpretive statements* (Fowler 2015, Provision 5; ICN 2021). Nurses often think of self-care as related to patients, no doubt because most of us learn Dorothea Orem's "Self-Care and Self-Care Deficit Theory" (Alligood 2018; McEwen and Wills 2017). From her theory we understand that everyone has needs that must be met; however, when the demand exceeds the resources we have or the capacity to meet them, then we experience a deficit. Nurses step into this deficit and try to either show the patient what to do, help the patient to do something of importance, or act to meet the need ourselves. These are important concepts in nursing, and they apply not only to patients but also to ourselves. Remember what flight attendants say when preparing people on an airplane for departure, emphasizing the importance of putting on our own oxygen mask first before helping those who need our help, because we must be strong enough and aware enough ourselves before we can be of use to others. It is through self-care that nurses will thrive rather than simply survive (Hill and Smith 1990).

SELF-CARE FOR NURSES

An American team of doctors and nurses (Baldoni et al. 2017) wrote a summary article on spiritual care in palliative care. They list eight areas of expertise, one of which is that health personnel should have training in self-reflection and self-care. Knowing how to care for yourself is crucial to avoid being exhausted and "burned out," when you could become vulnerable when in contact with other people's inner pain. This can be very demanding in healthcare service where we daily juggle many tasks and require-ments. In psychiatric nursing, for example, the nurse must rely on being able to effectively handle patients' unrestricted emotions. This means that a student or nurse is willing and able to accept and accommodate patients' unprocessed feelings, such as anger or frustration, without internalizing them. Being a self-care nurse is about being able to handle unprocessed emotion from the patient, by reasoning out what it means and giving it voice, because you understand that it is not about you as the nurse, but about the patient who is having trouble expressing and under-standing what is deeply felt (Schwartz et al. 2021). Some nurses can more easily do such an inner work and can respond to patient emotions in a way that the patient can understand and accept (Strand et al. 2017). Having compassionate care for self and our patients makes us open to others' grief, pain, and stress. So how can we manage to accept this without getting "stressed out" or having to shut down emotionally to protect ourselves? In addition to patient encounters, nurses also have work situations that we do not have complete control over, when there may be uncertainty associated with what happens on a shift.

When we become stressed, it affects our feelings causing us to become less tolerant and more irritable. It can also affect our thoughts so that we have less concentration and thus become less able to solve a problem. We will also notice the effects of stress on the body over time, because we can become tired and develop muscle tension, headaches, and nausea. In situations where we are under stress, it is important to think about what resources we have in and around us so that we can master the stress more effectively. The coronavirus pandemic has shown all of us in healthcare that we need strategies that can help us to alleviate the stress burden in order to stay healthy and avoid the many negative consequences of long-term stress (Blonna 2007).

We are responsible for caring for ourselves so that we can safely care for others (Fowler 2015; ICN 2021). We mentioned earlier that nurses are responsible for creating a welcoming and health-promoting work environment that demonstrates care for the employees, so a place where they can be seen and heard must be provided. We have also shown that journaling and using reflection groups are effective ways of dealing with challenging patient situations so that with our colleagues, we can understand situations better, develop new strategies for action, support each other, and become more effective in our patient care. We all need to be learners so that we can find new skills and approaches to self-care that will promote our health (Hill and Smith 1990).

SELF-CARE SKILLS AND STRATEGIES

This section deals with how each of us can take care of us ourselves so that we can train healthy and approachable students and nurses that patients can easily access. In Chapter 2, we wrote about how important it is to know yourself as a human being. Our reason is that each individual fills the nursing role with unique strengths and weaknesses, depending on who you are as a person. Having a deep inner motivation for nursing can provide a buffer against external stress. Knowing what is our foundation for hope and strength and what gives life meaning, we can search them actively to fight frustration and to replenish our own life. These foundations can be so many things. For some, it means to walk in nature, like the first author does when in Norway where there is walkway under a double row of trees that have been pruned over 100 years into a shape that resembles a cathedral archway. Walking there makes you feel like singing and praying! For others, it is to listen to certain types of music, to cook and bake creatively, or to spend time on various hobbies. For many, being together with the family and friends is a refreshing change from work and can be a real strengthening time. For others, it may be best to meditate or read poetry and other literature alone and away from busy people and constant noise. All of us have our unique ways of finding inner strength, and we need to schedule time in our busy lives for all of these uplifting activities.

Psychologists Anthony Schwartz and Barbara Wren (2012) report that it is important what resources and networks that each of us have around us and to what extent we understand the context of the system we work in so that we can cope with work related stress. Taking care of our own health is important in every area of life physically, emotionally, mentally, socially, and spiritually. In the physical realm, we must make sure that we eat healthy, sleep and rest enough, and engage in physical activity, because having a good balance between activity and rest is foundational to a healthy life. In addition, Schwartz and Wren (2012) recommend the following activities as part of good self-care:

- *Healthy self-awareness* is where we understand our own strengths, what stresses us, and what coping strategies we usually use. Recognizing how stress affects us cognitively, emotionally, psychologically and behaviorally can be important to understand when it is time to take specific steps to avoid burnout. It is important to learn to stop ourselves before we slide into negative feelings where we are just getting more and more tired.
- *Social support* means being able to talk with a friend, colleague, mentor, or supervisor that we trust and with whom we can freely share our experiences. Debriefing difficult situations with these trusted others can allow us to release tension and strengthen our inner self.

- *Letting go* means not to let the negative feelings build up within us, but to acknowledge what we feel and express what we experience verbally or in writing (personal journal). The example we gave earlier of using the "empty chair" activity to picture someone we wish we could talk to but cannot is a helpful means of letting go of our negative emotions.

- *Going on* means to follow our daily routines even when we are under pressure. Sometimes carrying out our normal routine helps us to regain perspective after a hard time.

- *Relaxing:* Don't eat or drink too much as a way of releasing stress; pause and take time to relax and do the things that help you relax and release tension. Listening to music, taking a fragrant bath, or using some form of meditation can help us to relax without causing harm to ourselves or others.

- *Analyzing* situations that lead to stress, and seeing if stress can be reduced, can be done using some of the strategies provided below (Blonna 2007). These activities can assist us by helping us to see what is triggering our stress. If it is internal stress, they can help us to take steps to master the situation; if it is external stress, then we can try to identify where more structural changes are needed in the work environment to reduce stress on those working in that space. It is good to consider an interdisciplinary approach whenever possible.

Reflection 5.2

- Reflect on the types of strategies you use to cope with stress
- What resources do you have to help you maintain a healthy balance in your life and work?
- In what areas do you think need more coping strategies?

American sociologist Richard Blonna wrote a very helpful book on *Coping with Stress in a Changing World* (2007) that describes how stress impacts the whole person. He makes the point that stress affects us physiologically, mentally, emotionally, socially, and spiritually, and that both the internal and external environment influence us and how we cope with the stress we encounter in our daily lives. Blonna describes "The Five Rs of Coping with Stress" that are very helpful:

1. *Rethink:* Changing the way you view things and their impact on you.
2. *Reduce:* Finding your optimal level of stimulation and changing for a better balance.
3. *Relax:* Using relaxation techniques [active and passive] to offset the effects of stress.
4. *Release:* Using physical activity (fun and laughter) to dissipate the effects of stress.
5. *Reorganize:* Becoming more stress-resistant by improving your health and prioritizing and focusing on what is most important first (Blonna 2007, p. vi).

For the first R – *Rethink*, you need to change your perspective on the world by examining your values, setting goals for yourself, slowing your pace, and enjoying life more (Blonna 2007, chapter 7). You also need to "rethink the way you view stressors" (2007, p. 186). Blonna looks at both Western and Eastern perspectives on thinking about stress, and he covers some interesting points on thinking about anger and road rage. For example, writing down your goals and prioritizing them, that is, naming them and ordering them by importance, can help you focus on positive elements and avoid self-anger if/when you do not meet your own expectations.

The second R – *Reduce* is about examining the stimuli and demands on us and their influence on us. We do this by (1) using the Three As of Coping (**A**bolish, **A**void, **A**lter – Blonna 2007, p. 209), which are discussed in more detail below (p.173), (2) identifying the demands on us, (3) managing them more effectively with the resources we have (2007, p. 210), (4) communicating more effectively (2007, p. 219), and (5) learning how to say no using the DESC Model (2007, p. 226), which suggests that we **D**escribe the specific situation, Express our concerns about it, State alternatives (attitudes, actions, conversations), and state the Consequences of letting things keep going in this way. In her work promoting a healthier workplace, Dr. Cynthia Clark (2015), a Fellow of the American Academy of Nursing, gives many good suggestions to promote civility, including a discussion of how to use the DESC Model in our conversations among healthcare personnel. This model is a good approach to assertiveness training. Clark believes that a healthy work environment requires "a shared organizational vision, values, and team norms; creation and sustenance of a high level of individual, team, and organizational civility; emphasis on leadership, both formal and informal; and civility conversations at all organizational levels" (Clark 2015, p. 2) because healthy workplaces will not evolve on their own; they must be developed and nurtured. Communicating clearly is a major key to reducing stress and its negative effects in our lives.

The third R – *Relax* has several important elements (Blonna 2007, chapter 9). First, Blonna compares the "stressed state" with the "relaxed state" (2007, p. 238), and then he encourages relaxation breathing (2007, p. 239) and meditation of various other types of passive relaxation (2007, p. 241). Meditation can use visualization (2007, p. 247) or guided imagery to increase a sense of peace. For

---

Box 5.2   Psalm 23

The Lord is my shepherd, I shall not want. He makes me lie down in green pastures; he leads me beside still waters; he restores my soul. He leads me in right paths for his name's sake.

Even though I walk through the darkest valley, I fear no evil; for you are with me; your rod and your staff, they comfort me.

You prepare a table before me in the presence of my enemies; you anoint my head with oil; my cup overflows. Surely goodness and mercy shall follow me all the days of my life, and I shall dwell in the house of the Lord my whole life long.

example, reciting, reading, or listening to the words from the 23rd Psalm (Bible, NRSV 1989) while picturing a lovely meadow with a gentle stream meandering through it can be very helpful and relaxing.

Other techniques that might be more active forms of relaxation include autogenics, which is a form of self-hypnosis using visualization and breathing together (Blonna 2007, p. 250), the "quieting reflex" and "calming response" (2007, p. 251) where you focus on the breathing itself, and biofeedback that uses equipment to monitor the physiological response to various relaxation techniques. Blonna concludes this chapter with a discussion of the use of hobbies, entertainment, and recreational activities that are fun and relaxing for us (2007, p. 253).

R – *Release* is the fourth way of coping with stress (Blonna 2007, chapter 10). Here, Blonna revisits the "fight or flight" response and then addresses the benefits of exercise and rigorous physical activity, such as dancing or kick-boxing. He describes the effects of mild, moderate, and vigorous activity, and finishes up with the cathartic effect of releasing stress even through something as useful as "mindful stove cleaning" (2007, p. 279). Blonna also touches on the release of stress through laughter, especially deep belly laughter, which he calls "a uniquely human reaction . . . indicating amusement, joy, or merriment" (2007, p. 278). In fact, he writes that:

> At least five major muscle groups react rhythmically when you laugh: the abdomen, neck, shoulders, diaphragm, and face. When you are finished laughing, they all are more relaxed than they were when you started. Laughter is a good tonic for muscle tension. (Blonna 2007, p. 278)

Maybe you can start a laughing club, like they have in some areas of India, or create a laughter diary that captures funny quotes or scenes, or even keep a stack of comic movies to watch when you need the release of laughter.

Finally, the fifth R – *Reorganize* addresses a way to become more stress-resistant. To do this, we must identify the path to optimal functioning and reorganize our life toward that goal. Blonna touches on how to address the environmental and occupational (workplace) as well as the social, spiritual, intellectual, emotional, and physical dimensions of health. Here the focus is on promoting health and wellness through positive coping strategies that can increase inner strength.

Reflection 5.3

- How do you feel stress in your body?
- What helps you release stress and refreshes you so that you don't "burn out"?
- What makes your heart sing?
- Identify at least two new coping strategies to try the next time you are feeling the burden of stress

AVOID BURNOUT

The words "burnout" and "compassion fatigue" are sometimes used interchangeably, but there are significant differences between them. Burnout is usually associated with the buildup of stress and tension from a variety of sources, while compassion fatigue describes what happens to nurses who have so much emotional burden that they become disconnected from their normal feelings when caring for patients and their families (Henson 2020). Compassion fatigue has been a problem during the current pandemic with the high volume of Covid-19 patients and the high death rate around the world (Gubbi 2021). There is a huge emotional toll on those who chose healthcare service in order to help people heal and/or successfully manage negative health conditions, but instead, they have ended up simply being present with many dying patients, which leads to high risk for compassion fatigue. We all need to share the burden of care among the members of the healthcare team, including the chaplains whose primary role is spiritual care (Speck 2014). Nurses and others in healthcare need to promote our own health by developing more coping strategies, which we address in the next section.

Burnout, on the other hand, has been a significant problem in nursing for decades (WHO 2019). The most effective way to avoid burnout in our challenging profession and stressful environment is to be proactive with understanding ourselves and developing positive coping strategies, as mentioned above. Build into your weekly schedule times of relaxation and refreshment so that you are strengthened and in a positive state of mind. It is a good idea to learn many coping strategies, even those that are not as interesting to you as some others, because we can pass them along to peers as well as nurse leaders who may have a wider influence in the workplace than we do. Prevention includes health promoting behaviors that are in the physical, mental (cognitive and emotional), social, and spiritual domains.

In the physical domain, most people know about the importance of physical activity for good health. Physical activity should be of a type that you enjoy; for some it is walking or jogging while for others it is dancing or using an exercise machine. Regardless of the type of activity, we all need to schedule it into our week. One thing not often mentioned is the importance of sleep and rest, which are very different things. Rest can bring relaxation and ease tiredness, but sleep is critical for renewal and restoration. Actually, deep sleep not only renews us physically, but if we actually go through all four stages of sleep (VeryWell Health 2021), then we can be psychologically and spiritually renewed through dream sleep. Good nutrition is also very important to keep in mind; we always tell our patients that we are each unique and have nutritional needs that must be met in order for us to have enough energy for our busy work lives. However, we often neglect to follow our own advice! Health promotion of our entire selves as nurses is the best way to care for ourselves and prevent illness and the feelings of being overwhelmed and "stressed out" at home and/or at work (Schwartz and Wren 2012).

Mental health is complex and challenging to promote (Medås et al. 2017) and must include strategies in both the cognitive and emotional arenas. We need to use things like self-examination and the "Five Rs" of Blonna (2007) to develop a repertoire of positive coping strategies before we become overwhelmed. Another helpful strategy is to use visual images that help us to focus inward and upward to whatever gives us strength. There are many helpful strategies and useful websites, as well as YouTube videos that can help nurses learn to cope with stress more effectively. The main thing is to remember that, while stress builds up cumulatively, stress reduction has a one-time effect unless you make it a regular practice.

The Center for the Contemplative Mind in Society (CMind 2021) encourages the practice of thinking meditatively and generatively through the visualization of a tree. You are the tree, and roots that are deeply buried in sustaining and nourishing soil are the foundation of life for you and for a deeper connection to the divine or transcendent. The branches include all types of practices, both quiet and meditative or active and generative, to help raise awareness, build inner strength, produce creative ideas, and increase coping skills (CMind 2021). We encourage you to consider visiting their website for a look at their Tree of Contemplative Practices: https://www.contemplativemind.org/practices/tree.

The social domain includes family and friends and social support of all kinds. In 1985, American nurse scholars Lyda Hill and Nancy Smith wrote the first nursing textbook on *Self-Care Nursing: Promotion of Health*, which is still relevant today (Hill and Smith 1990). They write that we need to promote health for ourselves in order to be strong enough to care for our vulnerable patients and to be safe while doing so. They note that nurses need to help each other and support each other in the workplace. We were created to live in community with others, so we need a sense of love and belonging in the world and in connection to others. Remember to nurture your supportive relationships. Build in time to be with those you love and enjoy. Don't neglect the deep friendships you have, or your spouse; it's too easy to assume that all will be well if we have a good marriage, but that can change if we fail to reach out to our partners/friends/family in the ways that they understand and appreciate. We also need to nurture our work relationships, especially in healthcare where we daily face hardships and suffering in our patients. In his wisdom writings from the Hebrew Bible, Israel's King Solomon reminds us of the *value of a friend* in the book of Ecclesiastes.

Box 5.3   The Value of a Friend

[9] Two are better than one, because they have a good reward for their toil. [10] For if they fall, one will lift up the other; but woe to one who is alone and falls and does not have another to help.

[11] Again, if two lie together, they keep warm; but how can one keep warm alone? [12] And though one might prevail against another, two will withstand one. A threefold cord is not quickly broken. (Bible, NRSV, Ecclesiastes 4:9-12)

It is always easier to face long shifts and difficult patient situations when we know we are not alone. We need each other! So, we need to communicate with and support our peers in the workplace. It is important for all of us to know that we have the support of our fellow nurses who truly understand what we are facing. So, spend time with each other, listen actively, engage attentively just like we try to do with our patients!

Spiritually, there are a variety of things we can do to help strengthen our inner spirits. Dutch ethicist Carlo Leget (2017) writes of the "inner space" we all have where we need nourishment and strength to face the challenges of today. This inner space is sacred space, not necessarily related to faith or religion, but it is the deepest place in our being, so it is special and precious, or sacred. Make time to do the things that nourish you there in your deepest heart, whether it is going out and spending time in nature, listening to your favorite music, or reading poetry, sacred literature, or the inspirational works of others. Schedule time each day for the things that enrich, refresh, and strengthen you. All of these things can help nurses to thrive and avoid burnout, but we need to keep on learning new strategies to help us cope more effectively.

DEVELOP COPING STRATEGIES

One of the most important ways that we can cope with stress is to pay attention to our bodies, minds, and spirits, and to know what is hard for us as well as what gives us inner strength. When we identify our stress triggers, we can use the "Three As" mentioned earlier to address them: *Abolish, Avoid,* or *Alter* (Blonna 2007). When possible, cut out contact with the person or thing in your life that causes that stress – *Abolish* it! Since that is not always possible, perhaps you can *Avoid* it, or you can *Alter* your way of thinking about that person or thing. For example, if there is always terrible traffic on your way to work, you might *Abolish* it by working virtually/online. Or perhaps you can change the route or travel time so that you *Avoid* such heavy traffic. If neither of those options is possible, you could decide to *Alter* its impact by spending the time in prayer (eyes open, please) and/or meditation so that you are refreshed within your spirit even though the circumstances of heavy traffic have not changed. Using these tactics can help manage stress of all types.

We can also use journaling and self-reflection to think about our life and what causes us to react or respond in the ways we do. It may be possible to confide in a close friend who can be a sounding board while we process our thoughts out loud. For some, this is more effective than journaling since some of us process things verbally and it helps us to hear what we are saying inside our heads and hearts! If we identify deep pain, it may be really important to go to a professional counselor to help us work through our memories or events in our past. Nurses are in a healing profession, and all health-care personnel need to remember to continually promote the art of healing, both for our patients and for ourselves (Jaiswal et al. 2019).

The coping strategies listed earlier that came from the work of Richard Blonna (2007) can add to our repertoire of strategies to use when facing stressful situations and/or people. The more ways we learn of how to cope with challenges, the more effectively we will use these strategies to help us live healthy lives in a constantly changing world. One thing to remember is that stress does build up over time, and it can contribute to the potential for burnout. Coping strategies, on the other hand, do not build up their effects. They do not stay and balance out the distress that we face in our day-to-day work and life; their effect is temporary and situational. Therefore, we need to build in or schedule in the strategies that help us cope! Schedule time for enough sleep and exercise, for meeting with social support networks, for helping us think more clearly and positively, and for being renewed in our inner space. Make room every day for the things that give you strength. For those with a Christian tradition, we remind you that Jesus told his followers, "Peace I leave with you; my peace I give to you. I do not give to you as the world gives. Do not let your hearts be troubled, and do not let them be afraid" (Bible, NRSV, John 14:27). Inner peace comes from being at rest within yourself, whether you have a faith tradition or not; it means keeping your inner sacred space clear of clutter and, instead, placing whatever refreshes and strengthens you there. This can help you handle all kinds of stress!

Reflection 5.4

Think about the domains of the physical, psychological, social, and spiritual self.

- In what areas do you feel the most stress?
- How can you increase your coping effectiveness in those domains?
- What activities can you schedule in that will help you thrive?

LEARN ASSERTIVENESS

In many places around the world, nurses have traditionally been taught to be submissive, but over the past 30 years, the feminist movement has made a difference in this view (McCabe and Timmins 2003). As our professional role has expanded, the need for assertive communication has increased. Nurses need to be assertive, not aggressive, when communicating with each other. Those within the Jewish or Christian traditions are familiar with the words of God to Joshua, the new Israelite leader after the death of the great leader Moses: "Be strong and courageous; do not be frightened or dismayed, for the LORD your God is with you wherever you go" (Bible, NRSV, Joshua 1:9). It takes courage to confront situations and people who are saying or doing the wrong thing, but if done assertively, good can result.

Again, kindness and courtesy should be our *modus operandi* so that we serve as role models to the entire healthcare team. Nurse leaders and educators must clarify the difference between assertiveness and aggressiveness so that students can learn effective ways to communicate difficult topics. We must all be supportive of each other, especially those who are new graduates or new to a specific healthcare organization. Instead of having a "nurses eat their young" reputation, let's promote courtesy, effective communication, and support for each other! Assertiveness training is very helpful if you feel like you cannot speak up at your place of work, so leaders should include it in further education for working nurses.

With assertive language, one thing we are reminded to use is "I" statements, so that we take ownership of our feelings when we feel threatened or "put down" at work. We can state in a non-confrontational way that when another person speaks in a particular manner or tone, or with specific words, we feel as though we are not heard or we are being put down. You can say, for example, "When you talk in that tone (or with those words), I feel anxious. I wonder if I have offended you in some way. Can you help me to understand what's going on here?" This opens up a conversation instead of burying our hurt feelings. We can also use this type of language to state our case: "I feel like my voice is not being heard and that my opinion is not valued. Can we clarify what is really going on here?" It is important for nurses to model our own value as a peer or employee, and for us to do our best to help promote a welcoming and healing environment for nurses and patients alike. In a real sense, we are using therapeutic communication techniques with each other, not simply with our patients. This will, hopefully, decrease the amount of lateral violence that nurses experience in our workplace.

MITIGATE BULLYING

It takes courage to confront bullying in the workplace. Lateral violence, or bullying has been on the rise in the twenty-first century, especially in recent years. Research from the National Health

Services (*NHS*) in the UK reveals that in 2001 there were some reports of "significant bullying," while in 2002 junior doctors experienced a 37% rate of bullying and nurses reported bullying at a 50% rate (Tim Field Foundation [TFF], 2021, section 7). Dr. Tim Field, who has done extensive research into bullying, identified several types of bullying:

1. *client bullying*, when one's patient and/or family applies pressure beyond normal anxious actions, or they verbally or physically assault healthcare personnel

2. *institutional/organizational/corporate bullying* in which the leaders foster an atmosphere where employees are pressured to work longer than normal hours or to carry a greater case load, workers are denied sick time or other normal benefits, or where they make it known that stress is only experienced by the weak and complaints about peers are encouraged

3. *serial bullying* by employees who have a pattern of obnoxious behavior that continues even if the recipient leaves their area of influence because they are dysfunctional and/or aggressive toward others in some way

4. *pair/gang bullying or mobbing*, where a group of people behave badly toward a peer, which usually happens when the institution ignores or even fosters this type of behavior

5. *secondary/residual/pressure bullying*, which is often unwitting and is due to stress causing the perpetrator to act in anger or some dysfunctional way, but who behaves differently when stress is relieved, or when the environment has a "zero tolerance" policy about bullying, and who can change if given guidance

6. *reactive/revenge bullying*, where the recipient of bullying responds with the same behavior or who later tries to pay back offensive actions they experienced

7. *peer/hierarchical/upward bullying*, the most common type in the healthcare environment, which involves negative

behaviors toward each other where the manager either joins in or refuses to tack action to stop the behavior and

8. *cyber bullying*, which is bullying at a distance through communication technology (Stopbullying.gov 2022).

Research findings on bullying caused many policy makers around the world to promote legal change and develop laws against workplace violence (TFF 2021). Currently, most institutions require employee training about harassment, whether sexual or some other type of bullying, to be done on a regular basis. Nurses need to stand together to support a "no tolerance" policy on bullying. The promotion of a welcoming and pleasant environment where such negative and offensive behaviors are not tolerated is up to both the leadership and the employees. Leaders need to ensure that training programs are followed and that negative actions have consequences. Nurse leaders need to foster an open mind with a kind response to employees' concerns. We should encourage employees to write any real concerns in a "grievance letter," promote a process of follow-up to any voiced or written concerns confidentially and quickly, and provide support groups where survivors can share their experiences and receive support and encouragement.

Employees need to take the required training, commit to positive and supportive behaviors with peers, and report situations where bullying is seen or experienced. Some recommended steps that can be taken are: (1) *regain control* by recognizing what is occurring in a specific situation and acting reasonably, (2) *plan for action* by learning about bullying and thinking through what is best to do in a variety of situations, and (3) *take action* by keeping a log of the negative behaviors and copying all electronic communication before going to a supervisor about the problem (Stopbullying.gov 2022).

Reflection 5.5

- Have you ever seen or experienced lateral violence or bullying?

- Think about that situation; ask yourself what you could do differently in a similar situation.
- What can you do to promote a welcoming and healing environment for you and your peers as well as your patients and their families?

WORKPLACE CARE: CREATING A WELCOMING AND HEALING ENVIRONMENT

We conclude by reminding our readers that it is up to nurses to make change in the profession of nursing. Spiritual care is never completely conquered; it is something we learn and grow in through life experience, educational programs, and a commitment to care for the spirits of our patients and those with whom we work. As lifelong learners, nurses can continue to grow both personally and professionally and to make a difference in spirituality and health for the good of our profession and the people we serve.

Practice self-care in your own nursing practice by paying attention to yourself and engaging in activities that will help you to thrive rather than just to survive. Determine what gives you inner strength, and practice activities that will do that, scheduling in time on a regular basis for your own spirituality. Learn to accept and like yourself and to be comfortable in your own skin. Learn to say "no" to things that will bring you down or exhaust you and send you toward burnout. Be sure to develop coping strategies; intentionally look for more ways to manage your stress. Find ways to deepen your personal spirituality and promote your health, and live fully and intentionally with an open heart.

Promote care for each other as nurses as well as for those around you, including leaders and other healthcare professionals. Be compassionate to all. A well-known biblical parable, "The Good Samaritan" (Bible, NRSV, Luke 10:25–37) was told by Jesus to remind his first century listeners that we should all treat each other as neighbors in this small world of ours, and that compassionate care is something we all need to give to those we encounter. In that story, a Samaritan, who at that time was considered a foreigner and enemy of Israel, found a Jewish man lying at the side of the road from Jerusalem to Jericho; the man had been robbed, beaten up, and left for dead. Three separate types of Jewish leaders took note of the man but passed by without helping. However, the foreigner stopped, cleansed the stranger's wounds with wine, soothed them with oil, and bound them up. The Samaritan man then put the wounded man on his donkey and took him to the nearest inn where he took care of him overnight and then paid for the man to be cared for while the Samaritan went on with his journey. Jesus asked his listeners who was a true "neighbor" to that wounded man, and the people responded that it was the one who had shown kindness and compassion. This is a great lesson for us all.

We encourage nurses to be kind and caring to each other, always giving the other person the benefit of doubt. Follow the advice of the Apostle Paul, a first-century pastor and community leader who wrote to his church at Ephesus, "Be kind to one another, tenderhearted, forgiving one another" (Bible, NRSV, Ephesians 4:32). This principle is true for everyone, regardless of whether you have a different faith or no religious tradition at all. Kindness and courtesy cannot be overrated in today's challenging environment. The poet Edgar Albert Guest (1891–1959) said it so beautifully in his poem on *Kindness* (Guest, 1956):

Kindness by E. A. Guest

One never knows
How far a word of kindness goes;
One never sees
How far a smile of friendship flees.
Down through the years,
The deed forgotten reappears.

One kindly word
The souls of many here has stirred.

Man goes his way
And tells with every passing day,
Until life's end:
"Once unto me he played the friend."

We cannot say
What lips are praising us today.
We cannot tell
Whose prayers ask God to guard us well.
But kindness lives
Beyond the memory of him who gives.

In addition to caring for each other, nurses need to help patients' families feel an atmosphere of warmth and welcome from us so that they are supported as they visit their loved ones. The first author remembers very well when her sister was extremely ill and a "spiritual care nurse" at a faith-based hospital took her out for a walk in the garden and encouraged her to trust in God and in the excellent care her sister was receiving. The nurse said that everyone who worked in that hospital was given a copy of the *10 Caritas Factors* of Jean Watson (Alligood 2018) on the back of their ID card as a reminder of how to interact with patients, families, and co-workers. How kind that nurse was, and what a wonderful experience of real care she gave!

One final word on spiritual care is that, just like with many things, "it takes a village"! We encourage you to consider being a role model for others by living and treating each other in positive, supportive ways. *Provide a welcoming and healing environment* for all. Build healthy relationships by being open, approachable, and honest so that other healthcare workers know they can trust you with their struggles. Never tolerate bullying or the attitudes and actions that diminish others; stand firmly and courageously against discrimination and meanness. Appreciate diversity and value differences; this will enrich your life! Encourage a sense of love and belonging by modeling genuine caring for your staff as well as patients. American poet Maya Angelou wrote, "I've learned that people will forget what you said, people will forget what you did, but people will never forget how you made them feel" (Angelou 2021, p.1). So, create a warm and healing environment by modeling positive ways of being with others. Be grateful for all that you have received and pay it forward by showing gratitude to all who work with you, for you, over you, and so on. An attitude of gratitude spread among each other goes a long way to strengthen support for each other and to promote healing. Be kind and forgiving, trust each other and give each other the benefit of doubt, and try to discern the healing path for those you serve (Puchalski 2013). Most of all, keep on caring for yourself and your own sacred space and for the deep inner spirits of all those who enter into your sphere of influence!

SUGGESTED RESOURCES

The Royal College of Nursing has a great resource: *Spirituality in Nursing* (RCN 2011), a pocket guide of the text that can actually fit in your pocket, though the print is small. You can find this manual by searching Google for the booklet title. It is a pdf: https://docplayer.net/16388491-Spirituality-in-nursing-care-a-pocket-guide.html.

   A Circular from the Norwegian Ministry of Health and Care Services: The right to one's own faith and vision of life refers to the court documents everyone who receives health and care tests in the municipality have to identify in order to facilitate exercising their own beliefs and life-views; you can find them most easily by applying for *Circular I-6/2009*.

   American Nursing Association documents like the *Code of Ethics for Nurses* (ANA 2015) and the policy statements (ANA 2010) can be accessed via https://www.nursingworld.org

   On YouTube there is a short presentation in English (6.30 minutes) on Viktor Frankl and his book *Logotherapy and Man's Search for Meaning*. Go to YouTube and search also for *Healing Spaces: The Science of Place and Well-Being* (mind–body connection) by Esther Sternberg

The author Emily Esfahani Smith has a TED Talk (12 minutes) about the difference between happiness and feeling. You find it by searching the web, either for its name or the title, *There is More to Life Than Being Happy* (https://www.ted.com/talks/emily_esfahani_smith_there_s_more_to_life_than_being_happy?language=en).

A number of movies offer insight into spirituality and how we can care more effectively for the spirits of our patients. See the classic movie *Patch Adams*, played by Robin Williams. This is a film depicting a true story about the medical student "Patch" Adams who challenges the medical profession by becoming acquainted with their patients and gaining insight into the dreams and the passions they have so that they can find the joy of life and the will to live. You can find a link to a short presentation of the movie by searching Patch Adams on YouTube.

In addition to the interview guides and suggestions for questions we have written about in Chapters 2, 3, and 4, there are a few other ways to do a systematic data collection that also includes the spiritual/existential aspects of patients. A "cultural formulation" interview in the DSM-5, NANDA – spiritual well-being versus spiritual distress – is useful, and the *Handbook of Religion and Health* by Koenig et al. (2012) can be found at Amazon (https://www.amazon.com/Handbook-Religion-Health-Harold-Koenig/dp/0195335953).

"Personal enlightenment, my life story" is a tool developed in *Aging and Health*, which shows various topics for the collection of information developed for persons with dementia or who have a problem with memory. You will find a link to this on the web by searching for "Personal Information, my life story." In addition, "Spiritual care in health care" by Peter Speck in the *Scottish Journal of Healthcare Chaplaincy* (Speck 2004) gives a good overview in brief.

Another work on the importance of critical reflection in healthcare practice offers a deep dive into this concept and contributes to personal meaning-making and spirituality (Hunt 2021). Just published by Palgrave Macmillan/Springer, the book addresses the concepts of critical reflection, transformative learning, vocation, and professional psychological well-being (https://www.springer.com/gb/book/9783030665906).

Online Resources

Many online resources are now available that can help both nursing students and working nurses. They can give inspiration for self-reflection and encourage our work with patients in relation to spiritual care. Some are provided throughout this handbook; others are listed below.

Bullying in Nursing

- www.bullying.co.uk/cyberbullying
- https://www.nursingald.com/articles/20231-discussing-the-unthinkable-bullying-in-nursing-and-healthcare

Creating a Healing Environment

- https://alska.com/2015/08/25/creating-a-healing-environment/
- https://scholarsrepository.llu.edu/cgi/view-content.cgi?article=1184&context=etd
- https://www.takingcharge.csh.umn.edu/creating-healing-environments-dr-esther-sternberg

Self-Care in Nursing

- https://www.purdueglobal.edu/blog/nursing/self-care-for-nurses/
- https://www.registerednursing.org/articles/ultimate-guide-self-care-nurses

EPICC SPIRITUAL CARE COMPETENCY SELF-ASSESSMENT TOOL

Spiritual self-assessment can be done using the tool found below. This self-assessment tool allows you to evaluate your level of knowledge, skills, and attitudes in four key areas of competencies for spiritual care. The tool was developed from the EPICC Spiritual Care Education Standard, which you can find on the EPICC Network website: www.epicc-network.org

Spirituality and spiritual care are understood as:

Spirituality: The dynamic dimension of human life that relates to the way persons (individual and community) experience, express and/or seek meaning, purpose and transcendence, and the way they connect to the moment, to self, to others, to nature, to the significant and/or the sacred. The spiritual field is multidimensional:

1. *existential challenges (e.g., questions concerning identity, meaning, suffering and death, guilt and shame, reconciliation and forgiveness, freedom, and responsibility, hope and despair, love and joy)*
2. *value-based considerations and attitudes (e.g., what is most important for each person, such as relations to oneself, family, friends, work, aspects of nature, art and culture, ethics and morals, and life itself).*
3. *religious considerations and foundations (e.g., faith, beliefs and practices, the relationship with God or the ultimate).*

EAPC (n.d.)

Spiritual care: Care which recognizes and responds to the human spirit when faced with life-changing events (such as birth, trauma, ill health, loss) or sadness, and can include the need for meaning, for self-worth, to express oneself, for faith support, perhaps for rites or prayer or sacrament, or simply for a sensitive listener. Spiritual care begins with encouraging human contact in compassionate relationship and moves in whatever direction need requires.

van Leeuwen et al., 2020

1. Please score yourself from 1 to 5 on each of the competencies, where 1 = Completely disagree, 2 = Disagree, 3 = Neither agree nor disagree, 4 = Agree, 5 = Completely agree.
2. Please write a short reflection at the end about your own competence in spiritual care.

Competency 1. INTRApersonal (within you) spirituality

Knowledge	1.	I understand the concept of spirituality	1 2 3 4 5
	2.	I can explain the impact of spirituality on a person's health and well-being across the lifespan for myself and others	1 2 3 4 5
	3.	I understand the impact of my own values and beliefs in providing spiritual care	1 2 3 4 5
Skills	4.	I reflect meaningfully upon my own values and beliefs and recognize that these may be different from other people's values and beliefs	1 2 3 4 5
	5.	I take care of my own well-being	1 2 3 4 5
Attitude	6.	I am willing to explore my own personal, religious, and spiritual beliefs	1 2 3 4 5
	7.	I am open and respectful to people's diverse expressions of spirituality	1 2 3 4 5

Competency 2. INTERpersonal (related to others) spirituality		
Knowledge	8. I understand the ways that people express their spirituality	1 2 3 4 5
	9. I am aware of the different world/religious views and how these may impact upon people's responses to key life events	1 2 3 4 5
Skills	10. I recognize the uniqueness of people's spirituality	1 2 3 4 5
	11. I interact with, and respond sensitively to, people's spirituality	1 2 3 4 5
Attitude	12. I am trustworthy, approachable, and respectful of people's expressions of spirituality and different world/religious views	1 2 3 4 5

Competency 3. Spiritual care: assessment and planning		
Knowledge	13. I understand the concept of spiritual care	1 2 3 4 5
	14. I am aware of different approaches to spiritual assessment	1 2 3 4 5
	15. I understand other professionals' roles in providing spiritual care	1 2 3 4 5
Skills	16. I can conduct and document a spiritual assessment to identify spiritual needs and resources	1 2 3 4 5
	17. I can collaborate with other professionals in the provision of spiritual care	1 2 3 4 5
	18. I can appropriately contain and deal with emotions	1 2 3 4 5
Attitude	19. I am open, approachable, and non-judgmental	1 2 3 4 5
	20. I am willing to deal with emotions	1 2 3 4 5

Competency 4. Spiritual care: intervention and evaluation

Knowledge	21. I understand the concept of compassion and presence and its importance in spiritual care	1 2 3 4 5
	22. I know how to respond appropriately to identified spiritual needs and resources	1 2 3 4 5
	23. I know how to evaluate whether spiritual needs have been met	1 2 3 4 5
Skills	24. I recognize my personal limitations in spiritual care giving and refer to others as appropriate	1 2 3 4 5
	25. I evaluate and document personal, professional, and organizational aspects of spiritual care, and reassess appropriately	1 2 3 4 5
Attitude	26. I show compassion and presence	1 2 3 4 5
	27. I am willing to collaborate with and refer to others (professional/non-professional) in providing spiritual care	1 2 3 4 5
	28. I am welcoming and accepting and show empathy, openness, professional humility, and trustworthiness in seeking additional spiritual support	1 2 3 4 5

This section is for you to reflect on your own competencies in spiritual care.

A. What are your strengths?

B. Which areas do you need to develop further?

C. How might you do that?

Note: Used with permission of the EPICC Network © EPICC Network 2021. Freely available on: www.epicc-network.org.

This self-assessment tool was developed from the EPICC Spiritual Care Education Standard, which you can find on the EPICC Network website: www.epicc-network.org.

REFERENCES

Alligood, M.R. (ed.) (2018). *Nursing Theorists and their Work*, 9ee. Mosby Elsevier.

American Nurses Association [ANA] (2010). *Nursing's Social Policy Statement: The Essence of the Profession.* https://www.nursingworld.org/practice-policy/nursing-excellence (accessed 22 March 2022).

American Nurses Association [ANA] (2015). *Code of ethics for nursing.* https://www.nursingworld.org/practice-policy/nursing-excellence/ethics/code-of-ethics-for-nurses (accessed 22 March 2022).

Angelou, Maya. (2021). Inspirational quotes on Amazon. https://www.amazon.com/Sincerely-Not-Inspirational-Angelou-Poster/dp/B07V5LH9MY/ (accessed 22 March 2022).

Attard, J., Ross, L., and Weeks, K. (2019a). Design and development of a spiritual care competency framework for pre-registration nurses and midwives: a modified Delphi study. *Nurse Education in Practice* 39: 96–104. https://doi.org/10.1016/j.nepr.2019.08.003.

Attard, J., Ross, L., and Weeks, K. (2019b). Developing a spiritual care competency framework for pre-registration nurses and midwives. *Nurse Education in Practice* 40: 102604. https://doi.org/10.1016/j.nepr.2019.07.010.

Baldoni, T.A., Fitchett, G., Handozom, G.F. et al. (2017). State of the science of spirituality and palliative care. Research part II: screening, assessment, and interventions. *Journal of Pain and Symptom Management* 54 (3): 441–453. https://doi.org/10.1016/j.jpainsymman.2017.07.029.

Benner, P. (1984). From novice to expert: excellence in power in clinical nursing practice. *American Journal of Nursing* 84 (12): 1480.

Bible (1989). *New Revised Standard Version [NRSV] of the Holy Bible.* National Council of Churches.

Blonna, R. (2007). *Coping with Stress in a Changing World,* 4ee. McGraw Hill: Higher Education.

Center for the Contemplative Mind [CMind] (2021). Tree of contemplative practices. https://www.contemplativemind.org/practices/tree (accessed 22 March 2022).

Cherry, K. (2021). The 4 stages of sleep. https://www.verywellhealth.com/the-four-stages-of-sleep-2795920 (accessed 22 March 2022).

Clark, C. (2015). Conversations to inspire and promote a more civil workplace. *ResearchGate* 10 (11): 1–7. https://www.researchgate.net/profile/Cynthia-Clark-/publication/302941121_Conversations_to_inspire_and_promote_a_more_civil_workplace_Let's_end_the_silence_that_surrounds_incivility/links/580b928008ae2cb3a5da6c5e/Conversations-to-inspire-and-promote-a-more-civil-workplace-Lets-end-the-silence-that-surrounds-incivility.pdf (accessed 22 March 2022).

Cone, P.H. (2020). An open journey approach to spiritual care education. *Atlas of Science.* https://atlasofscience.org/an-open-journey-approach-to-spiritual-care-education/ (accessed 22 March 2022).

Cone, P.H. and Giske, T. (2013b). Teaching spiritual care: a grounded theory study among undergraduate nursing educators. *Journal of Clinical Nursing* 22 (13–14): 1951–1960. https://doi.org/10.1111/j.1365-2702.2012.04203.x.

Cone, P.H. and Giske, T. (2018). Integrating spiritual care into nursing education and practice: strategies utilizing open journey theory. *Journal of Nurse Education Today* 71: 22–25.

EAPC (n.d.). EAPC Task Force on Spiritual Care in Palliative Care. https://www.eapcnet.eu/eapc-groups/task-forces/spiritual-care (accessed 18 February 2019)

EPICC Network (2021). Spiritual care educational Standard & Spiritual care self-assessment tool. http://blogs.staffs.ac.uk/epicc/ (accessed 22 March 2022).

Fisher, D., and Frey, N. (2013a). Engaging the adolescent learner. International Reading Association. https://keystoliteracy.com/wp-content/uploads/2017/08/frey_douglas_and_nancy_frey-_gradual_release_of_responsibility_intructional_framework.pdf (accessed 22 March 2022).

Fisher, D. and Frey, N. (2013b). The gradual release of responsibility model. In: *Better Learning through Structured Teaching: A Framework for the Gradual Release of Responsibility*, 2ee (ed. D. Fisher and N. Frey). Alexandria, VA: ASCD Copyright 2013 by ASCD.

Fowler, M. (2015). *Code of Ethics for Nursing with Interpretive Statements*. American Nursing Association.

Giske, T. and Cone, P.H. (2015). Discerning the healing path: how nurses assist patients spiritually in diverse health care settings. *Journal of Clinical Nursing* 24: 10–20. https://doi.org/10.1111/jocn.12907.

Gubbi, M. (2021). Kern County faces shortage in nurses due to Covid fatigue. *23ABC*. https://www.turnto23.com/news/local-news/kern-county-faces-shortage-in-nurses-due-to-covid-fatigue (accessed 17 September 2021).

Guest, E.A. (1956). Kindness. https://internetpoem.com/edgar-albert-guest/kindness-poem/ (accessed 22 March 2022).

Henson, J.S. (2020). Burnout or compassion fatigue: a comparison of concepts. *Medsurg Nursing* 29 (2): 77–95.

Hill, L. and Smith, N. (1990). *Self-Care Nursing: Promotion of Health*, 2ee. Appleton & Lange.

Hunt, C. (2021). *Critical Reflection, Spirituality and Professional Practice*. Springer.

International Council of Nursing [ICN] (2021). *ICN Code of Ethics for Nurses*. https://www.icn.ch/system/files/2021-10/ICN_Code-of-Ethics_EN_Web_0.pdf (accessed 22 March 2022).

Jaiswal, C., Anderson, K., and Haesler, E. (2019). A self-report of the Healer's art by junior doctors: does the course have a lasting influence on personal experience of humanism, self-nurturing skills, and medical counterculture? *BMC Medical Education* 19 (1): 443. https://doi.org/10.1186/s12909-019-1877-3.

Kelly, E. (2012). Competences in spiritual care education and training. In: *Oxford Textbook of Spirituality in Health Care* (ed. M. Cobb, C.M. Puchalski and B. Rumbold), 435–442. Oxford University Press.

Koenig, H.G. (2013). *Spirituality in Patient Care: Why, How, When, and What*, 3ee. Templeton Press https://doi.org/10.1177/0898010115580236.

Koenig, H.G., King, D.E., and Benna Carson, V. (2012). *Handbook of Religion and Health*, 2ee. Oxford University Press.

Kuven, B. and Giske, T. (2019). Talking about spiritual matters: first years nursing students' experiences of an assignment on spiritual care conversation. *Nurse Education Today* 75: 53–57. https://doi.org/10.1016/j.nedt.2019.01.012.

Leget, C. (2017). *Art of Living, Art of Dying: Spiritual Care for a Good Death*. Jessica Kingsley Publishers.

McCabe, C. and Timmins, F. (2003). Teaching assertiveness to undergraduate nursing students. *Nurse Education in Practice* 3 (1): 30–42.

McEwen, M. and Wills, E.M. (2017). *Theoretical Frameworks for Nursing*, 5ee. Lippincott Williams & Wilkens.

Medås, K.M., Blystad, A., and Giske, T. (2017). Åndelighet i psykisk helseomsorg: et sammensatt og vanskelig Tema [spirituality in mental health care: a complex and difficult topic]. *Nordisk Tidsskrift for Sygepleje* 31 (4): 273–286. https://doi.org/10.18261/issn.1903-2285-2017-04-04.

Puchalski, C.M. (2013). Integrating spirituality into patient care: an essential element of person-centered care. *Polskie Archiwum Medycyny Wewnętrznej* 123 (9): 491–497.

Ross, L. and McSherry, W. (2018). Two questions that ensure person-centred spiritual care. *Nursing Standard*. https://rcni.com/nursing-standard/features/two-questions-ensure-person-centred-spiritual-care-137261 (accessed 22 March 2022).

Ross, L., McSherry, W., van Leeuwen, R. et al. (2018). Nursing and midwifery students' perceptions of spirituality, spiritual care, and spiritual care competency: a prospective, longitudinal, correlational European study. *Nurse Education Today* 67: 64–71. https://doi.org/10.1016/j.nedt.2018.05.002.

Royal College of Nursing [RCN] (2011). *Spirituality in Nursing: A Pocket Guide*. London: Royal College of Nursing. https://docplayer.net/16388491-Spirituality-in-nursing-care-a-pocket-guide.html (accessed March 2022)

Rykkje, L., Søvik, M.B., Ross, L. et al. (2021). Enhancing spiritual care in nursing and healthcare: a scoping review to identify useful educational strategies. *Journal of Clinical Nursing* 2021: 1–25. https://doi.org/10.1111/jocn.16067.

Schwartz, A. and Wren, B. (2012). Caring for oneself. In: *Caring in Nursing. Principles, Values, and Skills* (ed. W. McSherry, R. McSherry and R. Watson), 16–32. Oxford University Press.

Schwartz, A., Baume, K., Snowden, A. et al. (2021). Self-care. In: *Enhancing Nurses' and Midwives' Competence in Providing Spiritual Care* (ed. W. McSherry, W. Boughey and J. Attard), 57–76. Springer Nature Switzerland.

Self-care in Nursing (2021). https://www.registerednursing.org/articles/ultimate-guide-self-care-nurses/ (accessed 22 March 2022) and https://www.purdue-global.edu/blog/nursing/self-care-for-nurses/?fbclid=IwAR0Vw9xGfX4Ff7j-yNo-EIQ5SqSxCjI_9lCPLkwYIL3A0fxi8kCW0LWJHUs (accessed 22 March 2022).

Speck, P. (2014). Spiritual care in health care. *Scottish Journal of Healthcare Chaplaincy* 7 (1): 26–30.

Stopbullying.gov (2022). What is bullying? https://www.stopbullying.gov/bullying/what-is-bullying (accessed 22 March 2022).

Strand, K., Carlsen, L.B., and Tveit, B. (2017). Nursing students' spiritual talks with patients – evaluation of a partnership learning programme in clinical practice. *Journal of Clinical Nursing* 26 (13/14): 1878–1886. https://doi.org/10.1111/jocn.13497.

Taylor, E.J., Testerman, N., and Hart, D. (2014). Teaching spiritual care to nursing students: an integrated model. *Journal of Christian Nursing* 31 (2): 94–99. https://doi.org/10.1097/CNJ.0000000000000058.

Tim Field Foundation (2021). "Bullying" (1996–2005 materials). https://www.bullyonline.org/old/workbully/nurses. html (accessed 31 July 2021).

van Leeuwen, R. and Cusveller, B. (2004). Nursing competencies for spiritual care. *Journal of Advanced Nursing* 48 (3): 234–245. https://doi.org/10.1111/j.1365-2648.2004.03192.x.

van Leeuwen, R., Tiesinga, L.J., Middel, B. et al. (2009). The validity and reliability of an instrument to assess nursing competencies in spiritual care. *Journal of Clinical Nursing* 18 (20): 2857–2869. https://doi.org/10.1111/j.1365-2702.2008.02594.x.

van Leeuwen, R., Attard, J., Ross, L. et al. (2020). The development of a consensus-based spiritual care education standard for under-graduate nursing and midwifery students: an educational mixed methods study. *Journal of Advanced Nursing* https://doi.org/10.1111/jan.14613.

VeryWell Health (2021). Health from A-Z: Trusted health information when you need it most. Know more, feel better. Accessed September 30, 2021 https://www.verywellhealth.com/.

World Health Organization [WHO] (2019). Burn-out an "occupational phenomenon": International classification of diseases. World Health Organization. https://www.who.int/news/item/28-05-2019-burn-out-an-occupational-phenomenon-international-classification-of-diseases (accessed 17 September 2021).

Further Readings

Cone, P.H. (2011). The Artinian intersystem model in nursing education. In: *The Artinian Intersystem Model* (ed. B.M. Artinian, K.S. West and M. Conger), 147–172. Springer Publishing.

Cone, P.H. and Giske, T. (2021). Hospitalized patients' perspective on spiritual assessment: a mixed-method study. *Journal of Holistic Nursing* 39 (2): 187–198. https://doi.org/10.1177/0898010120965333.

Giske, T. and Cone, P.H. (2020). Comparing nurses' and patients' comfort level with spiritual assessment. *Religions* 11 (12): 671. https://doi.org/10.3390/rel11120671

Haugan, G. and Rannestad, T. (2014). *Helsefremming i kommunehelsetjenesten* [Health promotion in the municipal health services]. Damm Cappelen.

Hovde Bråten, O.M. (2018). World views in Norwegian RE [religious education]. In: *Challenges of Life: Existential Questions as a Resource for Education* (ed. J. Ristineini, G. Skeie and K. Sporre), 147–176. Waxman Verlag GmbH. [Includes summary of *Lifeviews* by Aadnanes.].

McSherry, W. and Ross, L. (2002). Dilemmas of spiritual assessment: considerations for nursing practice. *Journal of Advanced Nursing* 38 (5): 479–488. https://doi.org/10.1046/j.1365-2648.2002.02209.x.

McSherry, W., Ross, L., Attard, J. et al. (2020). Preparing undergraduate nurses and midwives for spiritual care: some developments in European education over the last decade. *Journal of the Study of Spirituality* 10 (1): 55–71. https://doi.org/10.1080/204402 43.2020.1726053.

Medås, K., Blystad, A., and Giske, T. (2017). Åndelighet og åndelig omsorg i psykiatrisk sykepleie [spirituality and spiritual care in mental health]. *Nordisk Tidsskrift for Sygepleje* 31 (4): 273–286. https://doi.org/10.18261/issn.1903-2285-2017-04-04.

Okon, T.R. (2005). Spiritual, religious, and existential aspects of palliative care. *Journal of Palliative Medicine* 8 (2): 392–400. https://doi.org/10.1089/jpm.2005.8.392.

Pew Research Center [PRC] (2019). In U.S., decline of Christianity continues at rapid pace. https://www.pewforum.org/2019/10/17/in-u-s-decline-of-christianity-continues-at-rapid-pace/pf_10-17-19_rdd-update-new3 (accessed 22 March 2022)

Puchalski, C., Ferrell, B., Virani, R. et al. (2009). Improving the quality of spiritual care as a dimension of palliative care: the report of the consensus conference. *Journal of Palliative Medicine* 12 (10): 885–904. https://doi.org/10.1089/jpm.2009.0142.

Ross, L. (2006). Spiritual care in nursing: an overview of the research to date. *Journal of Clinical Nursing* 15: 852–862.

Skevington, S.M., Gunson, K.S., and O'Connell, K.S. (2013). Introducing the WHOQOL-SRPB BREF: developing a short-form instrument for assessing spiritual, religious and personal beliefs within quality of life. *Quality of Life Research* 22 (5): 1073–1083.

Van Leeuwen, R. and Schep-Akkerman, A. (2015). Nurses' perceptions of spirituality and spiritual care in different health care settings in the Netherlands. *Religions* 6 (4): 1346–1357. https://doi.org/10.3390/rel6041346.

World Health Organization [WHO] (2002). WHOQOL-SRPB Field test Instrument. http://www.who.int/mental_health/media/en/622.pdf (accessed 20 February 2019).

Index

The Nurse's Handbook of Spiritual Care, First Edition. Pamela Cone and Tove Giske.
© 2022 John Wiley & Sons Ltd. Published 2022 by John Wiley & Sons Ltd.